THE IMMUNITY SOLUTION

THE IMMUNITY SOLUTION

Seven Weeks to Living
Healthier and Longer

Leo Nissola, MD

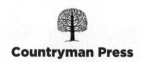

Countryman Press

An Imprint of W. W. Norton & Company
Celebrating a Century of Independent Publishing

Note to readers: The information presented in this book is the author's opinion and does not constitute any health or medical advice. The content of this book is for informational purposes only and is not intended to diagnose, treat, cure, or prevent any condition or disease. Neither the publisher nor the author can guarantee the complete accuracy, efficacy, or appropriateness of any particular recommendation in every respect.

Please seek advice from your healthcare provider for your personal health concerns prior to taking healthcare advice from this book.

To all survivors.

To Ivo and Ana, who dared me to be and
become, despite all adversities.

For Ben, whose love and support enabled my research, my
long working hours, and the publication of this book.

For Sandra and Brian,
whose resiliency inspires me every day.

For Padmanee and James, whose scientific breakthroughs
altered the course of human history.

To the light that enables our shared existence and
the love that binds us all together in life.

CONTENTS

INTRODUCTION

Cancer kills millions of people every year. It has taken loved ones from me, as with you and so many others. This biological bully—the emperor of all maladies, as Siddhartha Mukherjee beautifully describes it—reigns as a master of surprises, hitting when and whom we least expect.

By design, your immune system fights abnormal cells and prevents cancer, among other diseases, but over the course of your lifetime, it easily can sustain damage. Impairments can leave it struggling to fight diseases and leave you prone to illnesses. Today roughly 17 million people in America alone are living with cancer. Another 10 million Americans have compromised defenses, and at least 3.5 million suffer from an autoimmune disease. For some illnesses, the exact cause still remains unclear. We know that, for rheumatoid arthritis (RA), for example, the underlying mechanism involves the immune system attacking the joints. RA affects about 25 million people worldwide, but hard science about the disease's ultimate origins remains unknown.

When I was born in Brazil, President João Figueiredo ruled the country, the last in a series of dictators who came to power after a military coup roughly two decades earlier. In 1982, the year I was born, Swedish biochemists Sune Bergström and Bengt Samuelsson and British pharmacologist John Vane received the Nobel Prize in Medicine for their discovery of prostaglandins, a compound involved in inflammation reactions in the human body. Their research led to a new category of drugs that inhibit an enzyme called COX, which comes in two forms. The first affects the stomach lining specifically, and the second affects inflammation in general. Drug makers called this new group of non-steroidal anti-inflammatory drugs (NSAIDs). But the relief from inflammation and pain that NSAIDs afford comes at a high cost. Long-term use of NSAIDs can lead to gastric erosion, ulcers, and severe bleeding. So drug developers, wanting to target just inflammation, developed an NSAID called rofecoxib, which Merck sold as Vioxx. After regulatory approval, more than 80 million people took Vioxx.

A progressive disease, rheumatoid arthritis can lead to constant pain and swollen joints all over the body. It develops in phases, beginning with nonspecific inflammation, followed by chronic inflammation, and then tissue damage—in many cases severe. A few years after her RA symptoms started, my grandmother Maria's condition worsened quickly. She suffered terrible pain in her hands, wrists, and knees. The agony affected her mobility and led to hip and other joint replacement surgeries. In southern Brazil, where she lived, she didn't have access to a wide variety of frontline treatments. Apart from replacing the damaged joints, all her doctors could do was prescribe anti-inflammatories, including Vioxx.

Subsequent Food and Drug Administration (FDA) studies determined that taking rofecoxib led to an increased risk of death from heart attacks, strokes, and gastrointestinal bleeding. Before the manufacturer voluntarily took Vioxx off the market, it is estimated to have killed hundreds of thousands of people worldwide, including my grandmother. Once touted as a wonder drug, Vioxx became an abject failure of America's drug approval and oversight system.

My grandmother's painful, early death sparked my professional interest in immunology, autoimmunity, and drug development. My commitment to her legacy has pushed me to find safe ways to help heal people. I have dedicated my professional life to treating cancer and spearheading education efforts about the importance of a healthy immune system because the best way to cure cancer is to prevent it from occurring in the first place.

A decade ago, I began my research in autoimmunity, focusing on systemic lupus. Later I served as the lead physician for multi-billion-dollar drug assets at Johnson & Johnson as well as other top biotechnology and pharmaceutical companies. Working at the University of Texas MD Anderson Cancer Center, I met James Allison, PhD, who received the Nobel Prize in Medicine for his discoveries of negative immune regulations that led to new immunotherapy drugs to fight cancer. At the Parker Institute for Cancer Immunotherapy, I served as lead scientist for several early-phase clinical studies for patients with hard-to-treat, advanced cancers.

My life's work has required many sacrifices and difficult decisions. When my grandmother Maria died, I couldn't attend her funeral because I was taking my anatomy finals in medical school. When my other grandmother, Tereza, passed away, I was helping cancer patients at MD Anderson and couldn't travel to be with her in her final moments. When metastatic pancreatic cancer took my Uncle João, I was conducting trials for cancer patients at the Parker Institute during the darkest hours of the COVID-19 pandemic, when travel restrictions prevented me from saying goodbye in person. That's the price that other researchers and I pay for the work that we do and our commitment to give people a little more time to live their best lives and make beautiful memories. We don't want anyone to have to say goodbye sooner than necessary. Becoming an immunologist has felt not so much like a personal choice but like a critical mission to understand the complex interactions between our bodies and the external world.

In a twist of fate, at the same time that I was leading immunotherapy clinical trials, I diagnosed my own father with a rare immune-system cancer. Always in great health, he barely broke a sweat even when working hard. Then, out of the blue, in December 2020, he started having night sweats. He felt unusually fatigued. A few weeks later, just before Christmas, he video-chatted me to say hello. He sounded tired, and he looked skinnier than usual. I asked if he felt or noticed anything different recently. His description of how he felt immediately sounded like "B symptoms." In oncology, B symptoms indicate more advanced symptoms of cancer, which signify that the disease is systemic—spread throughout the body—and not localized in one specific area. Fevers, drenching night sweats, and an unintentional loss of more than 10 percent of body weight over 6 months all fall into this symptom category. With B symptoms present, the prognosis often looks grim because they forecast a high likelihood of metastasis, meaning that the cancer has spread.

I was in California, and my father was in Brazil. Thousands of miles and pandemic lockdowns separated us. Diagnosing a loved one with cancer is a doctor's worst fear, and all I could do was order lab work and scans and hope.

The test results confirmed the diagnosis I was dreading: metastatic lymphoproliferative neoplasia, a kind of cancer in which individual cells grow uncontrollably instead of into a single mass. But I had reason to be hopeful. Groundbreaking advancements in immunotherapy can help manage this particular cancer, and in his case they did. He's one of the lucky ones, his symptoms minimal because of the research that others and I have conducted. The drug combination he takes releases the brakes that stop some of his immune cells from destroying cancer cells.

But his diagnosis sounded an alarm for me to educate people about the power of the body's disease-fighting capabilities. Part of that mission is explaining how everyone can harness the power of the immune system and avoid these terrible diseases. I can't be everyone's doctor, but with this book I can show you how to strengthen your defenses so you can stay healthy, avoid disease, and live longer.

Your natural defense systems are nothing short of miraculous. While you go about your day and sleep at night, millions of immune-related processes are happening inside you that preserve your health and protect you from harm. By understanding your genetic makeup and the impact of your food and lifestyle choices, you can learn a lot about your body's ability to defend itself and what you can do to prevent yourself from getting sick. By taking a proactive approach to your health, you can improve your overall health, reset your immune system, and ward off future diseases.

This book contains a practical, science-driven, step-by-step guide (Part Three) to show you exactly what actions to take and what to avoid doing. Putting knowledge into action isn't always easy because it requires breaking certain bad habits, such as over-eating, excess stress, too much alcohol, and an unbalanced lifestyle. It also requires developing lifelong good habits, including eating better, sleeping better, calming your mind, and taking the right supplements when necessary. But the improvements in your well-being will make the journey worth it.

Good medicine stands on the shoulders of the latest science, and so does this book. When COVID-19 thrust the immune system into the international conversation, government officials, the media, and other organizations called on my expertise to help millions of people understand the science and guide them through it. This book will do the same for you, helping you see the link between your immune system and diseases that affect billions of people worldwide.

In this book, you'll find the keys to unlock the power of your immune system with my 7-week Immunity Solution Protocol, a 3-week immunity diet, and the practice of cellular feeding. With those guides, you can transform your health in just a matter of weeks, optimizing your immune system and fortifying yourself against the bacteria, viruses, and diseases that come into your life every day. When your immune system operates in top shape, it reduces inflammation in your body, which—bonus!—slows the aging process and can help some people lose extra weight.

Sometimes it takes a deep, personal loss to remind us that life isn't a spectator sport. That kind of pain changes who we are and shapes who we become. It has transformed me into a doctor with a message, an immunologist with a plan. Take stock of the loved ones you have lost and use their memories to summon the motivation to change your future.

Now let's get started.

PART ONE

YOUR BODY'S DEFENSES

1.

HOME TEAM:
YOUR IMMUNE SYSTEMS

"If you are not your own doctor, you are a fool."
—HIPPOCRATES OF KOS, the father of medicine

FIVE MINUTES REMAIN IN THE WORLD CUP QUALIFIER, AND THE SCORE stands tied. Two teams square off in center field. Everything is stacked against the underdogs: The weather is cold, the field is wet, this isn't their home turf, and they have less experience. But when the whistle blows and the ball flies into play, the underdogs hold a defensive line against the other, very aggressive team. The underdogs have what it takes to succeed, and because their team works well together, they win.

Your body's defense systems function a lot like that team. Different components serving in different roles all work together to help you fight a cold or even beat cancer. Hundreds of offensive volleys try to breach your body's defenses every day, but most of the time you stay healthy because your immune system prevents those invaders from making headway. Trillions of cells inside you constantly work to keep you safe. Every day they battle legions of bacteria and viruses. If your cells are strong, supported by your genes and good habits, they will win almost every battle. If they grow weak, trespassers can break through your defensive line, begetting cancer, diabetes, heart disease, and other illnesses. Maintaining a healthy immune system is the key to living longer and healthier. It works better than any miracle cream on the market, and best of all, it's already inside you. All you have to do is make good choices that support it, and it will do the rest.

Doctors know a lot about the immune system because it lies at the root of nearly everything that happens in the body. Luckily you don't need to have an MD to understand the amazing chemical interactions happening inside you, just as you don't need to be an electrician to use a lightbulb properly. But understanding how electricity works will help you understand which switch to flip.

WHAT IS THE IMMUNE SYSTEM?

Your immune system is your personal army. Think of it as a shield between your body and all the bacteria, viruses, and disease-causing pollutants in the world.

The most diverse system in your body, it consists of complex mechanisms that interact among cells, send signals, filter substances, and protect your tissues. Its purpose, though, is simple. It fights pathogens, which are disease-causing germs (bacteria, fungi, parasites, viruses). It removes potential threats from the body, such as splinters. It protects your body from potentially harmful substances, such as toxic chemicals. It identifies and neutralizes harmful substances in your bloodstream. It fights the effects of disease-causing chemicals, toxins, and cancer-causing agents. It prevents you from getting sick. If it can't contain a threat completely, it works to limit the damage.

Immunocompromised people have damaged or nonexistent shields that make them highly susceptible to everything, even the

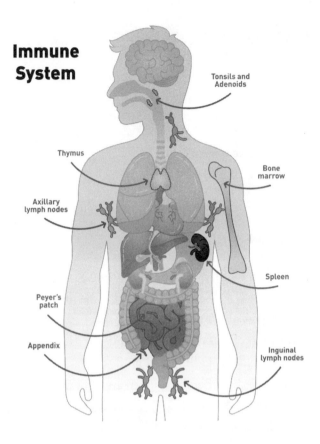

Immune System

Tonsils and Adenoids

Thymus

Bone marrow

Axillary lymph nodes

Spleen

Peyer's patch

Appendix

Inguinal lymph nodes

common cold. People living with cancer, uncontrolled HIV, systemic lupus, or genetic immune disorders can develop infections that people without those challenges don't. The same occurs in pregnant women, who naturally experience some immune deficiency during gestation. (Postpartum, their immune systems return to normal.)

The beauty of your body's natural defense system is that, as long as it's doing its job, you barely notice it exists. Sometimes, however, it can react aggressively to a perceived threat. When that happens, you can develop allergies or your immune system can attack normal cells, resulting in an autoimmune disorder. That's why it's so important to understand how the system works, what helps it work, and what doesn't.

WHERE IS THE IMMUNE SYSTEM?

It's everywhere in your body. These components all work together to form it:

- bone marrow
- complement system
- lymphatic system
- spleen
- thymus
- white blood cells

You probably have heard of bone marrow and white blood cells, but let's take a closer look at each of these parts of the system. Scientists believe that all immune cells originate from precursors in bone marrow, which produces white and red blood cells. White blood cells, like soldiers, fight infection. Bone marrow also contains stem cells, which can differentiate into a wide range of cell types, either to produce new cells or replace damaged ones. The complement system consists of proteins that help trigger inflammatory responses and fight infections. The lymphatic system, a network of small tubes running throughout your body, collects a fluid called lymph from your various tissues. The lymphatic system also collects dead cells and bacteria, and then it filters the waste through little bean-shaped nodes. Infections can cause lymph nodes to swell, sometimes resulting in pain in the neck, throat, or armpits. The spleen also fights germs, but its full function keeps broadening as scientists learn more about it.

Most people don't even realize that the thymus, a tiny organ, exists. Located in the upper chest, it matures your T cells, which your adenoids, appendix, gut, spleen, tonsils, and other places then store. Like your lymph nodes, the thymus helps remove pathogens and dead cells from your bloodstream.

AN EXTRA ORGAN

You probably can name most of the major organs—brain, heart, kidneys, liver, lungs, pancreas, skin, spleen, stomach, thyroid—but a lot of people don't realize that an "extra" one exists: the thymus. Unlike most organs, it's largest when you're a child because it's producing all your T cells before you hit puberty. As you age, it shrinks, replaced by fat. By age 75, the thymus essentially has become fatty tissue.

Your skin, a body-sized barrier, often serves as the first line of defense against microorganisms trying to invade your body. Healthy skin cells produce and secrete essential antimicrobial proteins. Immune cells gather in the skin's various layers because this organ plays such a vital role in protecting your body from chemicals, viruses, bacteria, and disease.

HOW THE SYSTEMS WORK

What happens inside your body every day is incredible. In the objects you touch, the air you breathe, and the food you ingest, you encounter countless potentially harmful organisms. All of them can make you sick, but usually they don't do anything to you because your immune system is doing its job.

Your immune system acts as your body's armed forces, your own personal Department of Defense. It has two main branches: the innate system and the adaptive system. Each functions differently in the ongoing quest to protect you. In simplified terms, you inherit your innate immune system from your parents, and your adaptive system develops throughout your life. Here's an easy way to differentiate the branches: The first relies on memory and the latter on specificity.

The Innate System

The second you're born, your innate immune system springs into action. Some people call it "natural" immunity because you have it from birth.

From your largest organ (skin) to your smelliest system (digestive tract), the innate immune system's cells serve as first-line heroes in the never-ending battle against potential threats. When your body sustains damage from an injury or germs, it triggers inflammation that recruits immune cells. The cells of the innate immune system arrive first, forming the body's initial line of defense. Innate immunity provides a broad, early bulwark against microbes, organisms so small that they're invisible to the eye and other pathogens, meaning anything that causes diseases and infections.

The innate system has many different types of cells, each with a specific purpose. These first-responder cells derive from stem cells in your bone marrow. White blood cells belong to this branch, as do other, more specialized cells that you might not know, including macrophages, mast cells, natural killer cells, and neutrophils. Some of these cells instantly attack foreign agents in the body, while others work together with other cell groups to prepare an attack. Like a soldier, each plays a crucial role in keeping you safe, but each plays a specific role.

Macrophages patrol your skin, mucus-bearing surfaces, and even your blood, looking for microbes. Macrophages derive from monocytes (explained below), but they don't circulate in the blood-stream. Instead, they operate in tissues. Macrophages absorb and digest pathogens found in their surroundings. When the immune system activates, monocytes and macrophages coordinate a quick

Immune Cells

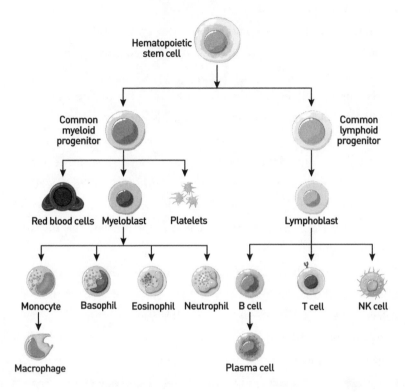

response by notifying other immune cells of a threat. Macrophages also recycle dead cells and sweep away cell debris.

Neutrophils, the most prevalent type of white blood cell, belong to the early-response team. They're your immune system's alert cells. They digest harmful cells and capture bacteria to prevent it from spreading. Because neutrophils circulate in the bloodstream, they constantly patrol the body for potential abnormalities. If you scrape your arm or bump your knee, neutrophils collect in the area within minutes. They communicate with one another, which allows them to coordinate and exchange signals with other cells. This cellular "swarm" calls macrophages and monocytes, which then surround the neutrophil cluster and establish a tight wound seal.

Monocytes, a type of white blood cell, can mature into macrophages or dendritic cells.

Phagocytes eat other cells, playing a crucial role in immune response by engulfing and destroying bacteria, viruses, and other threats.

Basophils, which circulate in your blood, play an important part in allergic reactions. As soon as these cells come into contact with certain antigens—short for antibody generators, meaning anything that triggers an immune response—they produce histamine, which attracts immune cells to the site. Your body responds by sending more blood to the area, generating inflammation in the form of redness, swelling, and warmth, which helps prevent the invasion from spreading further.

Mast cells, which operate in your tissues, also play a part in allergic reactions, helping the body defend itself against parasitic infections.

Eosinophils, like basophils, are kinds of white blood cells that help fight parasitic infections. They primarily attach to parasites too large to eat, essentially suffocating the invaders in order to kill them.

Dendritic cells are difficult to distinguish from monocytes. They present antigens, essentially showing other cells what to fight. Dendritic cells also break down large molecules into smaller, "readable" fragments (antigens) that B and T cells in the adaptive system can recognize.

Natural killer cells (NKCs), another type of white blood cell, function as the body's hunters. They recognize and latch onto aberrant bodies, such as viruses, chemicals, and cancer. NKCs consist of tiny compartments densely packed with proteins that they use to kill whatever is making you sick in a process called apoptosis, or programmed cell death. They eliminate targeted cells while causing limited damage elsewhere. NKCs work with both the innate and adaptive systems. They have the rapid response of innate cells but can accumulate biological memories like adaptive cells.

When a problem emerges, innate system cells respond swiftly and comprehensively, often causing inflammation. Problems with your innate immune system can cause chronic susceptibility to infection. Harmful microbes continuously evolve and change, trying to outwit your innate defenses. But your body learns from its experiences and develops ways to identify what belongs and what doesn't. The innate system can't do that on its own, though. As time goes on and situations change, your body needs upgrades, which is where the adaptive immune system comes into play.

The Adaptive System

This system creates and develops antibodies in response to germs the body previously has encountered. One of my virology professors cleverly calls the adaptive system "an acquired taste."

The adaptive immune system's cells constantly memorize and learn from germs and viruses in order to protect you even more. Memory in your immune system is vital. It allows for a faster response to threats and more efficient protection against antigens previously identified by your immune cells.

Your adaptive immune system develops from exposure to objects foreign to your body. That's one reason pediatricians encourage parents to allow babies older than 6 months to crawl around on the floor. Doing so brings them into contact with common household germs, which helps young children build antibodies. Studies have shown that sterilized environments and the overprescription of antibiotics make children less able to fight infections.[1]

The antibodies that your body develops from vaccines or run-of-the-mill colds all target specific strains. Collectively they improve your adaptive immunity.

Think of adaptive immunity like immune system boot camp.

INNATE IMMUNITY			ADAPTIVE IMMUNITY	
Eosinophil	Epithelial barrier	Mast cell	B cell	Antibodies
Basophil	NK cell	Neutrophil	Cytokines	Plasma cell
Dendritic cell	Complement	Macrophage	T helper cell	Cytotoxic T cell
HOURS			**DAYS**	

It gives your system information about other cells, prompting the adaptive system's cells to undergo thorough learning and training to fight new threats.

More specialized than innate immune cells, adaptive cells are called lymphocytes and fall into two groups: B cells and T cells.

B cells form in your bone marrow. Remember *B* for bone. Then they circulate throughout your body. When exposed to an antigen, a B cell becomes a plasma cell, or a living memory of how to tackle that microbe in the future. B cells alert T cells to the presence of a threat and deliver a one-two punch. B cells can evolve into cells that produce antibodies.[2] As soon as B cells recognize an antigen, they churn out antibodies that either destroy it or mark it as trouble. Those antibodies bind to the threat, making it easier for other immune cells to destroy it.

T cells also form in the bone marrow, but they migrate to the thymus to mature. Remember *T* for thymus. While T cells are

ANTIGENS

Any molecules that trigger an immune response are antigens. They can be anything: damaged cells, chemicals in infections, even the inanimate contents of dust. Adaptive immune cells identify antigens and respond accordingly, with the goal of preventing you from getting sick or sick again. For instance, if you had chickenpox or the chickenpox vaccine as a child, your adaptive system will recognize those viral antigens and prevent you from succumbing to the chickenpox virus (again). So not all antigens are harmful. A well-functioning immune system flags antigens it recognizes as normal and usually won't react against them.

growing in the thymus, they learn the difference between your own tissues and foreign objects. After maturing, T cells go through two selection stages to ensure that they don't bind to your own cells accidentally. Those stages protect your immune system from attacking you. Without them, you would suffer from serious auto-immune problems.

T cells can attack antigens directly. They use tools such as cytokines (explained below) to control and moderate the body's immune response. Usually, another immune cell, such as a dendritic cell, needs to break down an antigen so your body can recognize it, which triggers the process of making specialized T cells. Helper and killer T cells form the search-and-attack team for a particular antigen. Incredibly versatile, helper or regulatory T cells (Tregs) can tell your body when to stop responding to a threat and regulate its response. But when Treg function declines, disease can occur. An unwanted increase in Tregs can lead to cancer.

T Cell Activation

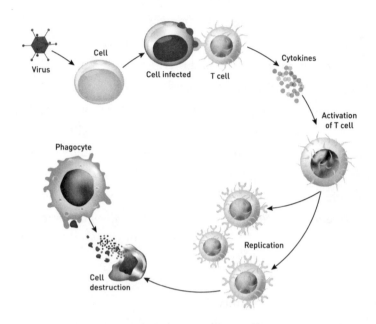

Lymph nodes serve as a communication center for immune cells, collecting information from the body. For example, if adaptive immune cells in a lymph node recognize fragments of bacteria from elsewhere, they will activate, reproduce, and leave the lymph node to attack the pathogen. The lymphatic system also acts as a conduit for immune cells. Depending on the pathway, your body can take days or weeks to acquire an adaptive immune response.

Natural, Artificial, and Passive Immunity

These three terms describe different kinds of adaptive immunities.

After you are exposed to and defeat an invader, long-lasting natural immunity occurs as a result. Your immune system leaves behind memory cells, which serve as physical reminders of what happened. It doesn't happen to everyone the same way because different factors, from diet to overall health, contribute to an immune response. Still, every time you have an immune reaction, your body takes notes. It might not always be permanent, but your body keeps track of past threats.

When you receive a vaccine, you develop artificial immunity. The vaccine activates immune cells that create a blueprint indicating how best to handle that pathogen in the future. Vaccines result in antibodies and memory cells that your adaptive system will call into service if and when a virus, such as measles or polio, or other germ tries to attack.

Passive immunity describes a situation in which immune cells come from a source other than your own body. It provides protection effective only for a short period of time, a few weeks or months. Fetuses absorb their mothers' antibodies via the placenta, and infants absorb them through mothers' milk, for example. Artificial passive immunity can come from injecting antibodies received from another person or animal. Treating snake bites with antivenom created by the snake is a perfect example of artificial passive immunity.

OTHER FIGHTERS

Several other supporting actors help your immune system in a variety of ways.

Toll-like receptors (TLRs) aren't cells. Proteins in the innate immune system, they span membranes, meaning they can enter cells from the outside. TLRs coordinate immune cell responses to microbes by signaling to the genes that need to respond. TLRs recognize patterns and a wide range of pathogens, including viruses, bacteria, fungi, and even noninfectious disorders. TLRs also bridge the innate and adaptive immune systems through dendritic cells.

Cytokines perform a variety of tasks, but mostly these tiny proteins serve as molecular messengers among cells. Some cytokines activate and focus the immune response by directing white blood cells to a certain location or showing them how to eliminate a specific bacterium. Cytokines also instruct your immune system to shut down after eliminating a threat.[3]

Interleukins are cytokines that deliver context-specific instructions that either activate or inhibit the immune system.

Chemotactic cytokines, or chemokines, are produced in certain areas of the body or at the site of an illness in order to recruit immune cells to come to the area. Different chemokines attract different types of immune cells to the required region.

Tumor necrosis factor (TNF) cytokines raise the inflammation flag, signaling to other cells to attack and kill invading cells. With diseases exacerbated by inflammation, such as rheumatoid arthritis, doctors prescribe TNF blockers to prevent this reaction. TNF blockers often treat various autoimmune diseases.

Antibodies, also known as immunoglobulins (abbreviated Ig), coat the surface of a pathogen and perform three key functions: neutralization, opsonization (coating it with proteins to enable a phagocyte to destroy it), and complement system activation. Memory cells in the adaptive immune system keep track of these antigens and the antibodies needed to fight them, and we call that process immunity.

IMMUNITY

Specialized cells of both the innate and adaptive immune systems create antibodies. Immunity happens in the body when enough antibodies fight or destroy a particular toxin or disease.

Antibodies are unique to a particular organism or set of organisms. They are created by the immune system in reaction to an infection and are unique to that particular infection.

Neutralization is the most common function of antibodies. A potential threat is neutralized when it is unable to connect to and infect host cells as a result of the antibodies that have been applied to it.

The complement system consists of proteins that interact to break down pathogens and trigger inflammatory reactions that help our immune cells to battle infection. Each protein triggers the next in a chain of events that continues indefinitely until the germ dies, is destroyed, or is marked for other cells to eliminate.

Interferons, a form of antibody, can inhibit or prevent a virus from replicating itself. Infected cells release these proteins, alerting nearby cells to imminent danger. Type I interferons provide antiviral responses, while Type II interferons generate antibacterial responses.

In simple terms, an immune response is your body's reaction to a threat, such as a splinter or a virus. Your immune system never sleeps. Always live, it actively defends your body 24 hours of every day. Complex and pervasive, it functions much like an army in which each cell has a specific function and task.

Allergic reactions and autoimmune conditions arise from unneeded or accidental immune responses. Infection or disease occurs when the immune response doesn't activate properly or at all. Carcinogens, chemicals, and other toxins can cause normal cells to malfunction and become unhealthy. Your immune system flags those damaged cells for removal. But when toxins overload the immune system, it can falter, which opens the door to disease, premature aging, and even death. That's why it's so important to do everything you can to optimize your immune system.

TAKE ACTION

- Pay attention to everything that interacts with your body on a daily basis: the hygiene products you use, the surfaces you touch, the food you consume, the liquids you drink, the air you breathe.

- Know the sources of the food, water, and personal care products you use every day.

- Wash your hands with plain soap for 20 seconds at least twice a day.

2.

GENETIC INFLUENCE: THE IMPACT OF YOUR DNA

"Genes are like the story, and DNA is the language that the story is written in."

—SAM KEAN, *The Violinist's Thumb*

IMAGINE A TEST THAT GAVE YOU ALL THE ANSWERS BEFORE YOU EVEN LOOKED at the first question. A test like that would have been pretty helpful in school. Today's genetic testing has become a modern cheat sheet for patients and healthcare providers. Spit into a tube or swab the inside of your cheek, pop the kit in the mail, and for as little as $99, you can gain access to information that ranges from your ancestral composition to your risk of developing certain diseases. Not all tests are equal, however, especially as more biotech companies see profit in offering these services. The company you choose matters. A quality test can deliver invaluable information that will provide a roadmap for ways in which you can grow old successfully.

Forewarned is forearmed, the old saw goes. Genetic technology can empower you to fight diseases before they manifest or to avoid passing problematic genes to your children. It gives you more accurate and more helpful information than whatever comes from the standard questions you answer about your family history on patient intake forms—especially so for adoptees who don't have access to their biological parents or family histories. Testing gives you and your doctors the tools to outwit your genes, if necessary, and to protect your future self from heart disease, diabetes, cancer, and hundreds of other conditions and diseases.

Every 30 seconds, someone in America receives a cancer diagnosis. That's two people in just the time it takes you to read this page. Right now, some 20 million Americans are fighting cancer, and another 1.2 million will join the battle this year. The best way to cure cancer is to stop it from developing, and the best way to treat it is also to prevent it from occurring.

That's why avoiding immune disruptors, knowing your biological age, and genetic testing are so important for staying healthy. Until now, modern medicine primarily approached illness by waiting for it to manifest and then attempting to treat it. All too frequently those treatments involved drastic, debilitating measures. You can get ahead of many life-altering illnesses by delving into your genetic code and taking charge of your health before it turns on you.

INSIDE YOUR DNA

Before we dive into genetic testing, let's recap a few concepts. Completely unique to you (unless you have an identical twin), your DNA contains all the instructions that your cells need to make proteins and other molecules essential for your tissues to develop, grow, and function properly.

Nucleotides, or chemical "letters," encode the basic recipe of your DNA. Like words on a page, the particular sequence of those letters—A for adenine, C for cytosine, G for guanine, and T for thymine—determines your genetic code and tells your cells what to do. Your body converts or translates the instructions built into your DNA into an RNA message. This message tells cells to produce strings of amino acids, which form proteins. The location of the letters determines the proteins' behavior, influencing how your cells operate and how your organs function. Think of it as a recipe written in another language. All the information is there, but it needs translating for the cells to perform the right step with the right ingredients at the right time.

Your cells read DNA sequences three nucleotides at a time, and each three-letter sequence, called a codon, specifies one amino acid. All protein-coding regions of your DNA begin with the sequence ATG, like a start button. Another three-letter sequence at the end functions like a stop sign or period at the end of a sentence. When you string it all together, each complete sentence forms a gene. Take the sentence, "The sun is hot." If that sentence represented a gene, your cells would read it like this: THE SUN ISH OT. The first three letters are the start button, the last three are the stop sign, and the letters in between contain the instructions for creating a particular amino acid.

AMINO ACID SPELLING BEE

Amino acids are the building blocks of proteins, which your body uses for growth, energy, and repair. Your body has 20 different amino acids that combine in different ways to create different proteins. If your DNA sustains damage that corrupts or removes one or more of those nucleotide letters, major disruption can result. Desert and dessert are two completely different concepts, separated by one little letter. Which one would you rather eat?

If letters shift, you can wind up in trouble. The phrase "HES UNI SHO T--" differs by just one letter from our example sentence, but that error, resulting from DNA damage, could lead to major problems. Consider a few real-world examples. Too much sun, smoking cigarettes, and exposure to toxic chemicals can cause DNA disruptions and alterations. When the letters and sentences become corrupt, just like a computer file, your body can't read the data properly and it malfunctions.

In the early 1950s, when scientists identified the double-helix structure of DNA, it became clear how the sequence of nucleotides encodes hereditary information in cells. Since then, subsequent researchers have made incredible progress toward understanding how DNA works. We have decoded entire genomes for many organisms, including—the goal of the Human Genome Project—ourselves.

NATIONAL DNA DAY

Congress designated April 25 as National DNA Day to celebrate two monumental achievements: the 1953 discovery of the DNA double helix and the successful completion of the Human Genome Project in 2003.

GENETIC TESTING

Understanding how genes, the full "sentences" of DNA, work will help you understand why genetic testing is such a valuable tool. When a sperm cell from your father fertilized an egg cell from your mother, the first cell of you formed. That cell contained the genetic blueprint for all of you, your entire body, from your hair to your toenails, including eye color and your potential risk for some ailments, such as asthma (often but not always linked to the ORMDL3 and GSDML genes).

As that cell divided and multiplied to form you as a fetus, a complete copy of the blueprint went into all the newer cells, much like copying computer files from one folder to another. Your muscle cells and liver cells, for example, carry out different tasks, but they still contain the same blueprints from that first cell. These are your inherited genes, which also contain the instructions for your innate immune system.

For decades now, doctors have been testing babies for genetic diseases. Virtually every child born in America undergoes mandated genetic tests to look for some 50 different diseases, including hypothyroidism, phenylketonuria, and sickle cell disease. This "heel stick" test enables doctors to undertake early-intervention treatments for the more than 3,000 babies who test positive each year.[4]

In adults, genetic testing makes use of blood, hair, skin, mucus, or saliva samples. Geneticists examine the cells in the sample and analyze your proteins, genes, chromosomes (the structures in your cells that carry your DNA), and even your biological age, which identifies the "real" age of your cells. Mutations and variations in your DNA can indicate diseases lurking in your body, such as Parkinson's, prostate cancer, or breast cancer. A variety of tests— DNA methylation age reports, proteome age profiles, inflammation markers, phenotypic age, and others—can help you measure the quality and capacity of your body's physiology, meaning your bodily functions. These tests give you a snapshot of what's happening or what might happen deep inside your body.

BIOLOGICAL AGE

Your epigenetic or biological age is how old your body thinks
it is. DNA methylation levels (the number of certain molecules
attached to your genes) measure your biological age. Social
factors, such as diet, drugs, environmental chemicals, hormones, and stress, can affect your DNA negatively. A buildup
of those methyl molecules can modify or interfere with the
function of your genes. If your biological age is higher than
your chronological age, your risk for many diseases increases
exponentially.

Regardless of whether tests come back positive or negative for
a particular gene mutation, having this information has potential benefits. Some common health risks, such as heart disease
and stroke, can pass down through families. Knowing the results
of those tests enables you to watch for and address risk factors.
Many couples undergo genetic testing to ensure they aren't passing genetic disorders to their offspring. These predictive tests can
provide relief from uncertainty and help you make informed
healthcare decisions. In some cases, negative results can eliminate
unnecessary checkups and screening tests, while positive results
can point you toward appropriate prevention, monitoring, and
treatment options.

Some people who learn that they're carrying the gene for a disease with no effective treatment can experience understandable
feelings of anxiety, depression, guilt, or rage. But a genetic test
can tell you only if you *carry* the genes. It can't predict accurately
whether you'll develop symptoms, the severity of the disease, or
its timeline.

It's never too early to become aware of a health problem so you can take steps to address it. You and your healthcare provider can use genetic insights into common health risks to create a personalized health plan to manage the onset of various conditions. These tests also can help you find out how much you've damaged your health already—or not—and potentially give you a plan to reverse the damage.

GENETICS AND YOUR IMMUNE SYSTEM

Contrary to popular belief, genetics aren't permanent. You can damage your DNA by excess UV exposure, drinking too much alcohol, consuming nicotine, and other means. Anything that compromises your immune system makes your body more vulnerable to chronic illnesses. It's like knocking holes in a brick wall. Eventually, the wall will fall because too much of it has sustained permanent damage.

Your DNA and immune system entwine. One affects the other and vice versa. After exposure to a threat, your immune system turns specific genes on or off to drive your body's overall response. Genetic factors also influence several types of immune cells, including monocytes, natural killer cells, and dendritic cells. Your genes determine much of your body's ability to defend itself, but everyday lifestyle choices are altering your genes, too. Genetics affects adaptive immunity more than innate immunity, and the environment affects innate immunity more than genetics. Those innate traits are the ones that, if you have children, you pass to the next generation.

Genetics preprograms your body's defenses, but your lifestyle choices can void that programming. Since 1965, the American government has required warning labels on cigarettes because their nicotine content and other carcinogens cause coronary artery disease. You could come from a family with no history of heart disease and no genetic markers for it, but if you smoke two packs of cigarettes a day, every day, you very likely will give yourself heart disease. Just because a bad genetic program isn't there doesn't mean that your lifestyle choices can't introduce it.

By that same token, just as you can degrade your health and immunity with poor diet and exercise, you can change the odds that your genetics have given you by making healthy choices that strengthen your immune system. Think of your body like a car. The more you expose it to extreme wear and tear, the more damaged it will become. But if you fill it with high-quality gas, do preventive maintenance, and give it regular tune-ups, the better it will run and the longer it will last. Preventing unnecessary wear and tear on your body is the backbone of my message because it gives you the keys to strengthen your immune system and to reverse the effects of aging, thereby causing you to live longer and better. A well-balanced life is the not-so-elusive secret of people who have lived past age 100.

Almost all chronic disease results from a complex interaction of genetic traits and environmental factors, meaning what you eat, what you drink, whether you smoke, how much you exercise, etc. Your risk for disease lies in the critical overlap between your genes

---

IMMUNE RESPONSE

Our bodies see every infection, illness, or disease as a potential mortal insult. Attackers can induce a natural response directly from our genes, which switch on or off to form the proteins discussed in Chapter 1 (page 7). We call this reaction the immune response.

---

and your environment. Understanding your genes empowers you to identify and modify nongenetic risk factors (smoking, drinking, eating, exercising, etc.), thereby lowering the probability you will develop many common diseases.

INFLAMMAGING

When any kind of threat—bacteria, toxins, trauma—injures your tissues, your body becomes "inflamed." Your body activates its inflammatory response when it detects the presence of certain chemicals in your body. Even extreme temperatures, hot or cold, can cause inflammatory reactions.

Ultra-processed foods, teeming with sugars, stabilizers, preservatives, emulsifiers, and artificial flavors, trigger inflammation. Combining those chemicals with seed and vegetable oils and other kinds of sugar can create even more inflammation. Examples of heavily processed food include store-bought bread, packaged cookies, protein bars, plant-based meats, lab-made eggs, and frozen dinners. Many vegan or plant-based products often contain anti-caking agents, artificial colors, artificial sweeteners, emulsifiers, mold inhibitors, and other toxic chemicals that aren't particularly healthy. Eat enough of those foods on a regular basis, and you put yourself at serious risk of developing inflammatory bowel syndrome (IBS).

When you experience inflammation of any kind, for whatever reason, your immune system springs into action. In some situations, the inflammation can result in DNA damage because too many defense cells heed your body's call and join the fight. Your immune system's one job is to defend your body, so when you introduce problematic chemicals, your immune system tells you to stop as often or as much as it encounters them. Those symptoms are a warning.

If your immune system thinks it's under attack, it will send an overabundance of white blood cells to defend you. They swarm to the rescue, but they have nothing to do and nowhere to go. Sometimes they attack your own organs or otherwise healthy tissues and cells, causing DNA damage. Those unwarranted attacks age your tissues, decay your overall health, and can lead to autoimmune conditions. Researchers call this reaction *inflammaging* (inflammation + aging). In addition to causing inflammation and accelerated aging, consuming ultraprocessed foods correlates with increased risks of developing cancer, cardiovascular disease, dementia, depression, kidney disease, metabolic syndrome, and type 2 diabetes. Researchers are examining the long-term implications of chronically consuming lab-made food. The inflammation created by this kind of diet can have whole-body consequences. If you eat something every day, that's a habit, and bad habits have significant consequences.

When your cells face near-constant attack because of that morning donut every day, those potato chips in the breakroom, or even the vegan "meat" you make for dinner, inflammaging can push your cells into senescence, or old age, meaning they stop multiplying and stop growing.

Cellular senescence initiates a cascade of negative immune responses, opening the door to (more) cancer, osteoarthritis, and other aging-related diseases. According to the latest research, cellular senescence is irreversible, and, like a runaway car coming downhill, it speeds the impact of any infection or disease that targets the body, including the severe acute respiratory syndrome (SARS) coronavirus, which causes COVID.

When your body's inflammatory responses are severe, your immune system may become less resilient, potentially lessening your ability to resist the effects of aging. In the COVID-19 pandemic, older adults, particularly those with preexisting medical conditions, showed an increased risk of experiencing uncontrolled inflammatory responses called cytokine storms. Many of those people died.

TELOMERES

Telomeres, or the little caps at the ends of chromosomes, can predict life span very accurately.[5] Like aglets, the tiny plastic caps on the ends of shoelaces or drawstrings, they help prevent tangling, fraying, or other damage.

When you're born, your telomeres are long and healthy because of telomerase, an enzyme present in sperm and eggs, blood cells, stem cells, and activated lymphocytes (B cells and T cells). In young and healthy people, telomerase continuously restores and extends telomeres. After you become an adult, the clock is ticking each time your telomeres shorten because they determine whether stem cells activate to regenerate and repair damaged or diseased tissues. Stem cells help maintain healthy

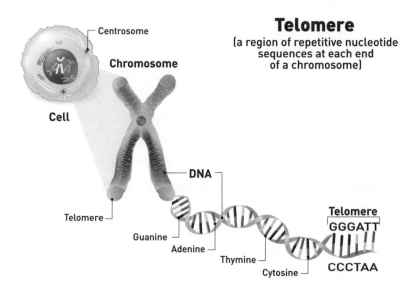

Centrosome

Chromosome

Cell

Telomere
(a region of repetitive nucleotide sequences at each end of a chromosome)

Telomere

DNA

Guanine

Adenine

Thymine

Cytosine

Telomere
GGGATT

CCCTAA

organ function, so a domino effect can accelerate the aging process. More about that below.

Elizabeth Blackburn, a postdoctoral fellow at Yale University, discovered the importance of telomeres in 1975 and received the Nobel Prize in Medicine in 2009 for her work. She realized that shortened telomeres indicate disease or aging. The shorter your telomeres become, the more susceptible your body becomes to damage and the faster you age.

Here's how the process works. Every time your DNA replicates during cell division—which happens 2 trillion times a day—a few nucleotides get "lost" in the shuffle, like a photocopier missing the last line of text on a page. These processes occur every single day, so what you feed your cells matters because they need good fuel to function properly. With each replication, DNA strands become shorter because your body can't replicate the tail end of your chromosomes. Telomeres, which are noncoding sequences, protect the strands from disappearing completely. They contain the same six nucleotides repeatedly. As your DNA replicates throughout your life, these repetitive sequences become shorter to protect the rest of your DNA. A human DNA strand runs about 3 billion characters long, so the process takes a while.

Imagine putting wet shoelaces through a hot dryer cycle over and over. The heat shrinks the fabric, making the shoelaces shorter. The heat also shrinks the aglets, making them cling more tightly to the shorter shoelaces.

Scientists think that this shortening of your DNA causes cells to age and causes you to age, too. Eventually the cells no longer can replicate, at which point they become senescent. Cells that reach senescence either accumulate damage or they die. DNA damage, as you might imagine, also causes telomere shortening. When the telomere unravels or "uncaps"—because the DNA has sustained too much damage to be repaired—programmed cell death (apoptosis) also can occur.

Telomere Shortening

Scientists are working on discovering the connections between telomere shortening and life span. Robust research has demonstrated a link between short telomeres and increased cancer risk—particularly bladder, esophageal, gastric, lung, and renal cancers—as well as diabetes, osteoporosis, and pulmonary fibrosis. For people between the ages of 60 and 75, individuals with short telomeres, compared to those with long ones, had at least a three times greater risk of dying from cardiovascular disease and a more than eight times greater risk of dying from infectious diseases. Telomere dysfunction also contributes to cellular exhaustion and impaired organ function. When they shrink, cells malfunction, organs begin to fail, and your health deteriorates.

Telomere shortening occurs naturally with aging, but accelerating that shortening can cause your cells to age more rapidly, thereby hastening the onset of various diseases. Researchers have seen telomere shortening in patients with chronic infections, in liver cells of people with chronic hepatitis, in intestinal cells of patients with chronic inflammatory bowel disease, and in patients with Alzheimer's disease. Telomere shortening can cause all kinds of complicated genomic instability (abnormal recombination, chromosome loss, and abnormal translocations). The shortening creates a domino effect: The shorter the telomeres become, the faster the aging process accelerates. The faster the aging process accelerates, the more your telomeres shorten. All of which raises an obvious question.

Protecting Your Telomeres

In medicine, knowledge is always the first step. Tests—over the counter (OTC) and from research institutes such as Johns Hopkins Medicine—can tell you the length of your telomeres. Some debate surrounds the accuracy of the OTC version, which costs about

$100. The test created in conjunction with Johns Hopkins costs about $400 and uses a different measuring method.[6]

These tests determine average telomere length by using peripheral blood cell samples and comparing the results with a database of people in the same age group. That data gives you a benchmark for whether you have telomeres shorter or longer than expected for your age.

Over brief periods, some natural oscillation occurs in telomere length. Researchers don't know exactly how much or whether the variation results from measurement errors or factors affecting daily behavior and health. If you do measure your telomeres, consider multiple tests to establish a reliable baseline.

If you want to stave off the aging process and avoid diseases such as cancer, then it makes sense to protect your telomeres. Their length at birth and the rate at which they shorten vary among individuals. Some people have abnormally short telomeres and experience accelerated shortening. But as you might expect, lifestyle and environment can have a significant impact on them. So the power to change them already lies in your hands.

Part Three of this book contains a more detailed plan, but here are the broad strokes:

- Avoid smoking.
- Avoid alcohol.
- Avoid ultraprocessed foods.
- Avoid processed seed and vegetable oils.
- Check your vitamin levels and supplement any deficiencies.
- Drink natural, mineral-rich water.
- Eat a nutritious, fiber-rich diet.
- Stay active.
- Maintain a healthy weight.
- Meditate.

Sound familiar? You've been hearing this medical advice for years because it all works!

Telomere Prescriptions

Along with lifestyle changes, certain medications can lengthen telomeres, including:

- angiotensin-converting enzyme inhibitors (ACEI)
- angiotensin receptor blockers (ARB)
- bioidentical hormone replacement therapy with aspirin
- calcium channel antagonists
- inhibitors of metformin renin
- antagonists of the serum aldosterone receptor

More research is necessary on this subject, however. As always, discuss any new treatments with your physician.

Lions, tigers, bears, and butterflies all rely on instincts to hunt better, run faster, or be more agile than their predators in order to survive. We humans, however, can outwit most of our enemies, including disease. That's why it's so important to understand how your body works, what decisions add wear and tear, and what actions can maintain your health. Applied knowledge, otherwise called intelligence, is the most powerful tool you have. Even if your genetic inheritance predisposes you to a particular disease, science has the tools to help you test, alter, mitigate, or even avoid your genetic destiny.

Aging is inevitable and you can't live forever, but as my father says, the joy of living should increase as we age.

TAKE ACTION

- If you haven't already, have your DNA tested. Learn whether you have any genetic predispositions to certain diseases or illnesses.

- Have you your epigenetic (biological) age tested.

- AVoid smoking, alcohol, and ultraprocessed foods, including processed seed and vegetable oils.

- Avoid unnecessary UV light exposure.

- Check your vitamin levels and supplement any deficiencies.

- Drink natural, mineral-rich water and eat a nutritious, fiber-rich diet of real, whole foods.

- Stay active and maintain a healthy weight.

- Meditate. If you can't do it every day, try for once a week.

3.

YOUR MICROBIOME: GOOD, BAD, AND UGLY GERMS

"Nothing in life is to be feared, it is only to be understood. Now is the time to understand more so that we may fear less."

—MARIE CURIE, winner of the Nobel Prize in Physics and the Nobel Prize in Chemistry

YOU MAY THINK THAT YOUR DNA MAKES YOU WHO YOU ARE. THAT'S PARTIALLY true, but it's not the whole story. DNA comes not just from your own human cells. It also originates from the countless bacteria that dwell on your skin, in your gut, and almost everywhere else in your body.

Even if you're not a germophobe, the idea that multitudes of other creatures live inside you feels a little creepy. But no human being is sterile, and that's good! Some immunologists argue that the world belongs to bacteria, and we humans are just living in it. These germs have inhabited the planet for more than 3.5 billion years, making them the oldest known life-form on earth, and you have nothing to fear about them. These microorganisms—bacteria, fungi, viruses, and other life forms inside you right now—want you to live because without you they'll die. They protect you in all sorts of incredible ways, from keeping gastric issues in check to fighting cancer. They form an entire world inside your body, collectively called your microbiome, and they play a critical role in training and developing major components of your immunity.

The overprescription of antibiotics, one of the hallmarks of modern living, has created the growing problem of bacterial resistance. We too often rely on medicines for quick fixes instead of trusting the natural systems inside our bodies to keep illnesses and diseases in check. By knowing how your microbiome works and how to take care of it, you can increase your immunity. Take care of these helpful microorganisms and they gladly will take care of you.

THE FUNDAMENTALS

It may feel nerve-racking to realize that millions of bacteria and viruses are keeping you company every day. But as one of my professors used to say, "No guts, no glory!"

Some are dangerous, even deadly, yes, but most help your health by maintaining balance. Some viruses, for example, live within you for your entire life without ever causing you any harm. They and their friends dwell in your microbiome, another of your body's systems that works in tandem with your immune system. Microbiota, a related term, indicates microorganisms in one particular area, while the microbiome refers to the big picture. Think of microbiota like a city and the microbiome as the whole planet. Some people use the two terms interchangeably, but for the purposes of this book, we'll use them properly: microbiota for a specific area, microbiome for the entire ecosystem.

The microbiome consists of approximately 100 trillion microorganisms. Microbes outnumber human cells by 10:1. You have more microbes in your body than cells. The main difference between the bacteria living on a doorknob, for example, versus what resides

MICRO VOCABULARY

Microorganism: A microscopic organism, often a bacterium, fungus, or virus.

Microbe: A microorganism, especially a bacterium, that can cause disease or fermentation.

Microbiota: Microorganisms located in one specific area.

Microbiome: The body's entire community of microorganisms.

---

in your body is that the majority of bacteria inside you is safe and probably good for you.

The first bacteria to colonize you came from your mother and have helped you stay healthy since birth. They came either from the birth canal or from your mother's skin in a C-section birth. These "good" microflora pass down through the generations and help early brain development. Breastfed babies receive additional immune strength though breast milk, which is rich in the good bacteria from the mother's body. Those first microbes in a newborn's gut break down the sugars in breast milk and set the stage for the rest of a person's life.

Most microbes enter your body via food and drink. They hang out in your digestive tract, usually the large intestine. All of them—bacteria, fungi, protozoa, viruses—contain genetic material that behaves just like your own genes. Because they're so small, you might think that they're pretty basic, but just the bacteria in the microbiome contain 200 times more genes than you have. Nothing survives for 3.5 billion years without packing a few unexpected punches!

Bacteria live and connect with your immune system in virtually every organ. They exist on the skin, inside the nose, in the mouth and throat, in the vagina, and primarily in the gut. Constant back-and-forth interaction keeps your body's immune system and those tenant microorganisms in check. Researchers continue to discover how the immune system and microbiome work together, including how different diseases can change the composition of the gut. That knowledge could enable us to prevent some diseases from occurring in the first place.

Bacteria on the Skin

Every day, your skin encounters toxins, hostile organisms, and other stresses. It acts as a physical protective barrier between your internal organs and the environment, yes, but it's also an active immune organ.

An estimated 20 billion T cells live in your skin, far more than in the rest of your body. Those immune cells ward off bad bacteria, fungi, and viruses before they can enter. Traversed by a network of blood and lymphatic vessels, your dermis—the medical term for the skin tissue beneath the surface—contains lymphocytes, leukocytes, mast cells, and macrophages. Why so many different kinds? If you get a cut, even a little one, any bad bacteria on the surface of your skin (the epidermis) can make their way inside. Puncture wounds are even worse, creating oxygen-free portals straight into your body.

Remember, your body constantly patrols for foreign invaders. Tattoos survive because immune system cells in your skin eat the ink and pass it to the next generation of cells. Studies show that tattoo pigment can undergo successive cycles of capture and release without fading, which creates a constant immune response. The components of tattoo ink are mostly manufactured, so not natural to the body, but nanoparticles from the ink can travel throughout the body, causing lymph node enlargement and allergic reactions. That's a lot of unnecessary labor for the immune system just for a pretty picture. I have four tattoos. I don't regret them, but if I could go back in time and talk to my teenage self, I would say: skip the tattoos.

Bacteria in the Body

In the gut, bacteria help you digest food, protect your intestines from foodborne pathogens, and create vitamins, such as B_{12} and K, which your body doesn't otherwise produce. Most people have a good balance of more than 1,000 different types of bacteria. They come in different shapes and sizes and fulfill different functions. Many aid digestion, but they also can serve as an early protection system.

When you eat, you introduce lots of new bacteria into your mouth. The good bacteria already there will kill a lot of the bad guys, and regular brushing and flossing will remove the sneaky, stubborn ones that survive. If that balance tips in bad bacteria's favor, then bad breath, gingivitis (swelling of the gums), cavities, tooth decay, and even heart disease can result. That's right,

---

TETANUS

The tetanus vaccine—which all school-age children receive and adults should receive as a booster every 10 years—prevents the development of lockjaw. That disease can result from exposure to the tetanus bacteria, which loves the low-oxygen environment of puncture wounds. (It has nothing to do specifically with rust, a common misconception.) The bacteria cause the muscles to tighten in terrible spasms, which proves fatal in about 10 percent of diagnosed cases. The tetanus shot boosts the immune system to fight that bad bacteria.

---

not taking care of your mouth can lead to bad bacteria in your bloodstream, which can harm your heart. Halitosis is your body's way of telling you that something isn't right.

GUMS AND HEART HEALTH

A 2014 study from the *American Journal of Preventive Medicine* found that people with gum disease spent 10 to 40 percent more on cardiovascular care.[7] Estimates put the risk of gum disease affecting your heart at 20 percent, and additional research shows links between poor oral health and respiratory illnesses, osteoporosis, and cancer. Oral diseases cause inflammation, and chronic inflammation anywhere overtaxes your immune system, allowing other diseases to take hold. So brush, floss, and see your dentist regularly.

Other diseases, such as obesity, IBS, and diabetes can develop when you ingest too many processed sugars, fats, and chemicals instead of natural, beneficial foods, such as vegetables. Veggies contain prebiotics, a fancy word for compounds that help your good gut bacteria flourish. (More about prebiotics shortly.) People who develop these diseases usually have lower-than-normal percentages of good bacteria in their guts.

Bacteroidetes: The Good Guys

These bacteria grow in soil, fruits and vegetables, seawater, humans, and other animals. A balanced population of bacteroidetes busily produces metabolites that help reduce inflammation in your body. A high-fiber diet can increase their number, while a low-fiber diet reduces your body's ability to respond appropriately to inflammation, particularly the kind caused by allergies in the lungs.

Firmicutes: The Bad Guys

These not-so-cute bacteria heavily populate the gut. When they outnumber their good counterparts, firmicutes can impair the metabolism of glucose and fat. Some studies have found that an increased ratio of firmicutes correlates with a rise in obesity and type 2 diabetes. Having too many firmicutes can unbalance your metabolism and energy levels. Immunologists believe that the bacteria that make people more prone to obesity are draining their bodies of energy, which makes them even more susceptible to obesity-related health conditions.

The Gut-Brain Axis

Scientists increasingly refer to the human gut as the body's second "brain" because it contains approximately 100 million neurons, more than the spinal cord or nervous system combined.[8] Those neurons control many reflexes, including the secretion of enzymes to help break down food and the contraction of the muscles that aid in digestion.

Bacterial Happiness

During stressful situations, that knot or dropping feeling in your stomach is a conversation between your brain and gut. Serotonin, the "happy hormone," sends messages to cells that help regulate emotions and happiness. But contrary to popular belief, this neurotransmitter comes mostly (about 90 percent) from your gut, *not* your brain, and it greatly influences gut immunity.[9] It also helps maintain body temperature, aid digestion, and improve blood flow, breathing, and sleeping.

Gut-Brain Axis

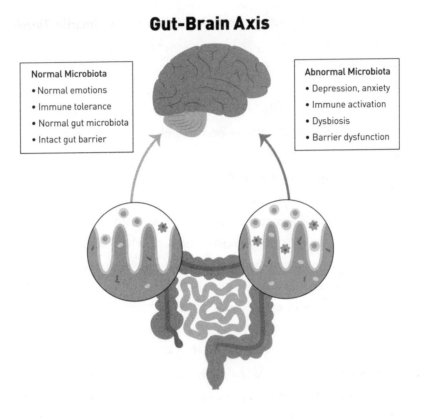

Normal Microbiota
- Normal emotions
- Immune tolerance
- Normal gut microbiota
- Intact gut barrier

Abnormal Microbiota
- Depression, anxiety
- Immune activation
- Dysbiosis
- Barrier dysfunction

TRUST YOUR GUTS

The neurons that connect your mind and gut communicate more than just hunger. They trigger the sensation of butterflies when you feel nervous or anxious, or a tightening when you feel scared. The lesser-known enteric nervous system runs through your whole digestive tract, from esophagus to anus. It uses the same network of neurons and neurotransmitters as the central nervous system and plays a significant role in mental health and other disorders. The science about this connection continues to form, but it's always a good idea to heed whatever messages your body is sending you.

One study showed that a mixture of bacteria, primarily *Turicibacter sanguinis* and *Clostridium sporogenes*, signaled gut cells to increase production of serotonin. Laboratory mice raised without those bacteria had 50 percent less serotonin than a control group. When researchers added the missing bacteria to the deficient mice, their serotonin levels increased to normal.[10]

THE MICROBIOME AND THE IMMUNE SYSTEM

Pediatricians encourage parents to let their babies crawl around on the floor. That activity not only teaches little ones about surfaces, smells, and the sensations of depth and gravity, but it also introduces them to lots of microorganisms. This early exposure helps build babies' immune systems.

At peak performance, the gut has its own active immune system that protects you from unwelcome viruses, chemicals, and other environmental factors. When poor choices or good intentions disrupt your system's balance, disease can result much more easily. Those good intentions refer to what researchers call a hygiene hypothesis. The theory holds that extreme personal hygiene has led to an increase in diseases because of reduced exposure to natural, friendly microbes. In essence, we're washing, sanitizing, and medicating away all of our body's natural fighters. If you don't break a major sweat, you don't need to shower every single day. Every other day is better for your skin and your immune system.

Drugs and modern science help us fight diseases, but consuming synthetic foods and excessive antibiotics, among other bad habits, harms the diversity of disease-fighting bacteria in your microbiome. That imbalance puts your body in a weaker position when serious threats approach. It's like pulling half of a defensive army out of battle before the invading army doubles its forces. The defending soldiers won't be able to defend the castle, let alone push the invaders back.

WELCOME TO THE VIROME

Viruses are the most common biological entities on earth, and you have more of them inside you than you probably know. At least 38 trillion bacteria inhabit your microbiome along with 380 trillion viruses.[11] They coexist with you peacefully and beneficially most of the time. Some of them even kill bad bacteria, preventing you from getting sick.

Pathogens can take advantage of poorly managed microbial environments and grow uncontrollably. This opportunistic growth can cause serious inflammation because the body's immune guards have deactivated or simply aren't there. That's why gut dysbiosis can prove so damaging to your overall health.

Bacteria versus Cancer

Some gut bacteria trigger inflammation and even cancer. Researchers have been trying to identify the mechanisms that allow cancer to develop in epithelial cells, for example. With colon cancer, no single bacteria species is always responsible. But it's possible that that kind of epithelial cancer results from a shift in the types of gut bacteria.

At the same time, scientists are examining bacteria to see whether they can cure cancer. At the Parker Institute for Cancer Immunotherapy, I conducted an early-phase clinical trial trying to answer one question: Can gut bacteria help patients with advanced melanoma fight the cancer?

We already know that an unbalanced microbiome allows diseases to take hold. An increase in gut permeability may allow nutrients, minerals, and salts to leak and penetrate other layers, leading to inflammatory disorders such as rheumatoid arthritis and type 1 diabetes. Patients with a good gut balance respond better to immunotherapy, so we theorized that the right gut bacteria could serve as a new immunotherapy tool. This study that I helped design, write, conduct, and evaluate was one of the first of its kind.

My colleagues and I partnered with leading institutions and experts across America to test our hypothesis. The clinical trial examined whether altering the gut microbiome of cancer patients could enhance or otherwise change their responses to immunotherapy. Before, during, and after immunotherapy treatment, we sequenced the guts of all participating patients to analyze changes in their tumors and track changes in their immune systems. The COVID-19 pandemic unfortunately forced us to discontinue the study, but subsequent evidence suggests that our hypothesis was correct.

DAMAGE AND DIVERSITY

Your gut manages a powerful symbiotic relationship between the rest of your body and the creatures that help digest your food and keep the pipes clean. Don't think of all the bacteria that live in and on you as invaders but beneficial extensions of your body. Upsetting that balance can create a dysfunctional environment.

When disease-causing microbes build up in the body over time, they alter metabolic processes and genetic activity, triggering abnormal immune responses. New research appears to indicate that autoimmune diseases pass down through families not strictly through DNA inheritance but also through the transmission of the family's microbiome.[12] You can reset your microbiome, as you'll see in Part Three of this book, but first you should know what factors damage it. Then you can work on repairing and strengthening it.

Imbalance

Scientists call bacterial imbalance in the body, particularly in the gut, dysbiosis. It interferes with your body's normal workflow, predisposing you to obesity, IBS, and in some cases even colorectal cancer. Mounting evidence shows a clear connection between dysbiosis and increases in diabetes, fibromyalgia, metabolic diseases, multiple sclerosis, muscular dystrophy, obesity, rheumatoid arthritis, and other conditions. It remains unclear whether dysbiosis contributes to the development of these diseases or correlates with their precursors, but the link still worries metabolic researchers.

Many factors can lead to dysbiosis, including environmental impoverishment. Yes, you read that last sentence correctly. A lack of diversity in the gut microbiota can start on a global scale and eventually affect individuals. Ecological degradation takes place when habitats, predator populations, and the biodiversity of animals and plants all shrink. Polluting the planet, clear-cutting rain forests, and building strip malls decrease diversity across the board. The resulting domino effect can reverse evolution and move life backward into less complex, stable states. Scientists believe that damage on a macro level correlates with a decline in good bacteria in your microbiome.

In the last few decades, many immune-related diseases have become more common. This rise happened first in Western countries and has spread more recently to developing nations. These diseases include allergies, inflammatory bowel diseases, metabolic disorders, type 1 diabetes, multiple sclerosis, and colorectal cancer.

Immigrants to Western countries more likely develop many of these illnesses, especially if they move before age 5, which points to the impact of early environmental risk factors. What happens in the world at large can mirror what's happening inside your body. One influences the other, in positive and negative ways. Changing the world can change your health and vice versa. How can you do that on a personal level? Respect and protect local habitats. Don't let your pets kill local fauna. Support local farms. Buy organic. Plant local, pollinator-friendly flora. Reduce, reuse, recycle.

Other origins for dysbiosis include poor diet, broad-spectrum antibiotics, alcohol use, and bad dental hygiene. The good news there is that, also on that personal level, you can control or modify most of those considerations by eating healthily, taking antibiotics judiciously, ditching antibacterial products that contain triclosan or triclocarban, reducing or eliminating your alcohol intake, and looking after your mouth—all of which means reversing the damage to your microbiome.

Also, not all dysbiosis is bad. For instance, fecal transplantation works well to treat people suffering from *Clostridium difficile* colitis or type 2 diabetes. Medicine's next big breakthrough might just be understanding the unknown connections among the different systems in your body and the diseases trying to take hold in them.

PREBIOTICS AND PROBIOTICS

First, a note on terminology. Prebiotics, foods typically high in fiber, help your existing gut microbiota thrive. Probiotic foods contain living microorganisms—the good bacteria—to help restore balance to your system. In recent years, both have surged in popularity, making their way into foods, pills, and even beauty products. But they're not all (created) the same.

YOGURT CULTURE

Ilya Mechnikov, winner of the Nobel Prize in Medicine, proposed that aging results from bacterial toxins in the gut and that lactic acid–producing bacteria can slow the aging process. In a 1905 lecture, he linked microbes in sour milk to the longevity of Bulgarians, setting off an immediate, international spike in the demand for yogurt.[13]

Probiotics can improve your health by displacing potentially harmful bacteria. But the benefits apply only to a small number of conditions, and the market for them has little regulation. They don't have to work in order to be sold, and quality control can be lax. Packaged probiotics don't help as much as natural foods, and some can cause infections in people with weakened immune systems.

Between 2016 and 2017, the FDA inspected more than 650 facilities manufacturing dietary supplements, finding violations in more than half of them. The infringements included concerns about products' purity, strength, and even identity. The facilities were manufacturing a variety of supplements, including probiotics and prebiotics.[14] Some probiotic supplements contain unwanted

BETTER BIOTICS

Good prebiotics: garlic, onions, leeks, asparagus, dandelion greens, seaweed.

Good probiotics: kefir, yogurt with live active cultures, sauerkraut, tempeh, kombucha, kimchi, miso.

organisms. Supplement contamination is thought to have resulted in the death of an infant in 2014.[15]

The best way to incorporate prebiotics and probiotics into your diet is to eat natural, organic foods.

SEX AND THE MICROBIOME

From birth, your hormones influence your microbiome. Unless you alter your natural hormones, they continue to affect your gut microbiota throughout your life. Sex hormones potently determine the types of bacteria in your body. In adolescence, when sex hormone production blossoms in earnest, microbiological differences between males and females also manifest. Changing estrogen levels propel girls into womanhood, while steady testosterone levels propel boys into manhood.

Some health disorders don't seem sex specific, but, for instance, more women than men receive diagnoses of clinical depression. People with depression have different microbiomes than people who don't suffer from that malady. Some gastrointestinal disorders, such as IBS, affect women twice as much as men. Children identified as male at birth are more likely to receive autism spectrum diagnoses, and, you guessed it, their gut bacteria differ as well. Oscillations in the amounts or proportions of those hormones—which naturally exist in all of us—could explain why women have a more diverse and more changeable microbiome than men. It's also possible that immune responses differ between men and women because of these varied microbiomes.

If it all sounds a little deliriously complicated, that's because it is. Just keep listening. Life is every bit as complex as the systems that maintain it.

TAKE ACTION

- If you have tattoos, give your immune system a break by not adding more to the mix. If you don't have any tattoos, keep it that way.

- Make sure your tetanus booster is up to date.

- If you have a crawling-age baby, let him or her explore the floor (while keeping an eye out for choking hazards).

- If you don't break a significant sweat, shower every other day.

- Respect and protect local habitats. Don't let your pets kill local fauna.

- Support local farms and buy organic.

- Plant local, pollinator-friendly flora.

- Eat healthy. Incorporate asparagus, dandelion greens, garlic, kefir, kimchi, kombucha, leeks, miso, onions, sauerkraut, seaweed, tempeh, and yogurt with live active cultures into your diet.

- Avoid unnecessary antibiotics and antibacterial products containing triclosan or triclocarban.

- Listen to your dentist and take good care of your mouth.

4.

BROKEN LINKS: WHEN THE SYSTEMS GO AWRY

"Everything can be taken from a man but one thing: the last of the human freedoms—to choose one's attitude in any given set of circumstances, to choose one's own way."
—Viktor Frankl, *Man's Search for Meaning*

BUSY MODERN LIFE SEEMS SO IMPORTANT UNTIL SOMEONE YOU LOVE OR YOU yourself get sick. When your system malfunctions, you quickly understand that nothing matters more than your health. Most of the time, your immune system works as it should, defending your body against invading organisms, pollution, and chemicals. But not always.

A broken genetic link, the development of a devastating illness, or a sudden reaction can cause the whole system to misfire. Immunologists see it every day in patients with autoimmune disorders and immunodeficiencies. Autoimmune conditions often are described as rare, but they're not uncommon. Type 1 diabetes, hypothyroidism, and multiple sclerosis affect between 14.7 and 23.5 million people in America alone, almost 10 percent of the population. The autoimmune category includes more than 80 conditions, many of them chronic and debilitating, such as rheumatoid arthritis.

Before COVID-19, more than 6 million people worldwide were dealing with long-term immunodeficiencies.[16] As doctors learn more about long COVID, those numbers probably will rise. The medical community already is seeing an increase in immunity issues after exposure to the SARS coronavirus that causes it. Immunodeficiencies can leave you vulnerable to new infections and put you at risk for developing autoimmune disorders, cancer, and other diseases. Deficiencies result from an impaired immune system. In autoimmune disorders, the immune system attacks itself. The stronger your system, the stronger the attack. That's why you need to strengthen your immunity but also optimize it.

AUTOIMMUNE DISORDERS

When the immune system attacks proteins in its own tissues, autoimmunity occurs. With autoimmune disorders, your body's early warning systems can fail, or your immune cells can misfire. Not all immune disorders result from genetic causes, and not all autoimmune diseases are created equal. Some genetic components may underlie the disorder, but they aren't always the main cause. Some autoimmune disorders result from infections, others from exposure to chemicals, and yet others from dietary choices. For those reasons, many people develop immunity disorders later in life. These illnesses don't discriminate when it comes to age, ethnicity, income, or even celebrity status. It's easy to manage some autoimmune disorders. Others become a lifelong battle.

Everything—the air you breathe, the food and water you consume, the personal hygiene products you use, the environment around you—impacts your health now and down the road. When your body encounters too many chemicals or your microbiome becomes unbalanced, your defense systems can malfunction, resulting in many of the issues discussed in this chapter. In the last 30 years, the number of diagnosed cases of autoimmune disorders has doubled in America.[17] Researchers point to specific chemicals, including mercury, pesticides, and cigarette smoke. Many socio-economic variables also relate to the continued increase, including chronic overexposure to microplastics, lead, arsenic, and other hazardous chemicals.

One study, published in 2007, shows a tragic example of how chemical exposure can impact the immune system and cause disease. It examined a spike in lupus cases in a housing subdivision built atop a defunct oil field in Hobbs, New Mexico.[18] The oil field closed in 1967. Developers built the subdivision in 1976, and remediation efforts had been in place since 2000. The oil company had installed a vapor recovery system and a tank battery to reduce storage tank vapors. Still, residents in a six-block radius regularly noticed a rotten-egg smell in the air and black oil oozing from their yards. The number of lupus cases in this area was 30 to 99 times higher than in the general population.[19]

A quarter of the study participants had detectable blood levels of pristane, phytane, or pristanic acid. All of the people with those chemicals in their blood also had immune system disorders. When researchers analyzed their blood samples, they noticed a significant difference in the number of B cells and natural killer cells. This community didn't just have a higher-than-normal number of lupus cases. Residents also had far more neurological, cardiovascular, respiratory, and gastrointestinal issues. All from an operation that had ended four decades prior. This kind of data underscores why it's so important to limit your exposure to harmful chemicals.

Doctors don't know the exact mechanisms by which chemicals lead to autoimmune disorders, but the connection is crystal clear.[20] Toxins can cause your body's warning systems to malfunction and put them on high alert. When that happens, your immune system targets cells contaminated by the chemicals, creating autoimmunity. In the Hobbs, New Mexico, study, residents encountered those chemicals in the air they breathed every day and in the yards where their kids played—years of constant contamination exposure every time they drank a glass of water or mowed the grass.

Here's another example from my life. One Sunday, a friend called me in a panic. She woke that morning to find clumps of hair on her pillow. More chunks of hair fell out as she was showering. She preferred natural items to processed or packaged versions, and she didn't eat much meat. She hadn't had any recent operations or hospitalizations, although she had been feeling "different" lately. Her health seemed fine until a few months earlier, when some strange symptoms developed. She felt drunk after just one glass of pinot noir. Her hair, never chemically treated, became lifeless and brittle. She felt nauseated and lightheaded for no apparent reason. She coughed sporadically, almost as though she had developed new allergies. She never had had bronchitis before. She complained of dry skin all over her body, accompanied by mild anxiety.

I sent her to see a trusted immunologist. She didn't meet the traditional criteria for lupus, which meant additional testing. She saw a rheumatologist, an allergist, and even her gynecologist. After that extensive medical tour, she felt more confused than ever. The specialists didn't rule out an autoimmune condition, but they didn't confirm it, either. She did test positive for every marker of inflammation, however.

It turns out that her health problems had begun 6 months before she called me, when she moved into her new house. She subsequently had her water tested and learned that it contained more than 20 cancer-causing chemicals. They entered her body every time she took a drink, cooked a meal, brushed her teeth, bathed, or washed her hair. Her new home stood just a couple of miles from an oil refinery. She didn't have an autoimmune disease. She had toxic water.

As I explained to her, when the immune system attacks healthy tissues in our bodies, inflammation results. It can cause joint and skin problems, even organ failure, along with pain, fatigue, and other nonspecific symptoms. With most autoimmune illness, the symptoms appear so similar to other ailments that many people endure long periods of misdiagnosis. Recent research indicates that receiving a correct autoimmune disease diagnosis in America takes more than 4 years and nearly 5 doctor visits.[21]

Autoimmune disorders are so variable that it's difficult even for specialists to identify them properly unless they deal with them on a daily basis. Even then, it can prove a challenging road to navigate. Laboratory testing, clinical assessments, and a battery of exams help distinguish autoimmune disorders from other diseases. Common auto-antibody tests, while useful, can cause even more confusion if performed incorrectly.

Chemical intoxication isn't the only cause of autoimmune diseases, either. Imbalanced microbiota can impair your intestines, which normally stop most invading pathogens in their tracks. A vicious circle then forms. A compromised gut, when hit with exposure to toxic chemicals, becomes weaker and less effective as the exposure continues.

People with autoimmune disorders have a variety of treatment options that include medication and dietary changes. That's right: According to growing research, what you eat can help regulate inflammation and autoimmune responses. Many disorders, including hypertension, cardiovascular disease, and strokes, correlate closely to consuming excess salt and polyunsaturated fatty acids (PUFAs).[22] For years, the medical and nutritional communities have advised people to avoid saturated fats and instead to choose unsaturated fats, which is good advice, but you should avoid nonanimal fat altogether in favor of easily processed, animal-derived fat.

Recent research has revealed that gut microbiota play a meaningful role in a variety of disorders, including type 1 diabetes, irritable bowel disease, and obesity. Gut microbiota also may affect central nervous system illnesses, such as multiple sclerosis.[23] Those microorganisms influence not only the gut environment but also the body's overall immune responses by changing the balance of pro- and anti-inflammatory cells. Diet modification might represent the most promising treatment strategy in the context of autoimmunity.

AUTOIMMUNE CONDITIONS

Autoimmune disorders cause your defense cells to respond abnormally to normally functioning cells, which can harm any tissue or system in the body. These disorders are chronic, systemic, and sometimes severe. Scientists don't fully understand these situations in which the body's immune system misfires and destroys its own tissues. I've been studying them for more than a decade, and I still have more questions than answers because no two autoimmune patients are alike, either.

Many public figures have shared the details of their autoimmune disorders. Pierre-Auguste Renoir, a founder of the impressionist style of painting, had one of the first well-documented cases of rheumatoid arthritis. The condition left him wheelchair-bound for the last 20 years of his life. Even so, he painted through his pain by tying the paintbrush to his hand. More recently actors such as Tatum O'Neal and Kathleen Turner have gone public about their battles with rheumatoid arthritis, which often leaves them painfully exhausted. Lady Gaga has struggled with lupus.

NOT EVERYTHING IS GENETIC

A world-class dermatologist once diagnosed me with psoriasis, an autoimmune disorder, swearing that my case was genetic and that I couldn't do anything about it. Psoriasis can run in families, but I refused to accept his doomsday diagnosis. Instead, I stopped smoking, and the disease completely went away. Later research revealed a link between smoking and psoriasis.[24] Not all cases are genetic. Some result from lifestyle choices. Yet another reason to quit smoking or not to start in the first place.

Let's take a look at a handful of the more common diseases along with some of the luminaries using their platforms to shine light on those illnesses.

Lupus

Like many autoimmune disorders, lupus is a difficult condition to define and diagnose. It has vague and variable symptoms, it can appear and disappear without warning, and the severity of the symptoms can range from minor discomfort to death. Researchers have identified no one gene or set of genes as responsible for the disease. When it appears in families with no prior history, no one knows why. Nor are any two lupus cases alike. It develops when antibodies meant to fight infections attack the body's own tissues.

Approximately 90 percent of diagnosed lupus patients are women, particularly between the ages of 15 and 45. African Americans, Hispanics, and Asian Americans are more likely to develop lupus. It occurs most commonly in women of color. African American women are more than three times more likely than Caucasian women to have it. The disease proves more common in African

Americans than in West Africans, indicating that social, dietary, and environmental factors play a crucial role in its development.

Some people have a predisposition to lupus, which infections, certain medications, or even sunlight can trigger. A complex combination of genetics, social circumstances, diet, chemical exposures, and the environment probably causes it, but we don't yet fully understand how. We do know that pesticide exposure correlates to an increased risk for developing the disease. People with an inherited predisposition may develop the disease if they come into contact with a trigger, such as food, drugs, or chemicals. In the vast majority of cases, the root cause remains unknown. Sun exposure can trigger a flare-up in someone who already has it, but we don't know if the sun alone is the culprit or if it affects the disease because of prior chemical exposure.

Most people with lupus have a mild form of the disease marked by flares, meaning that symptoms worsen for a period before improving or even disappearing completely. The most distinguishing symptom is a facial rash that looks like butterfly wings unfolding across both cheeks. This rash occurs in many but not all cases. Symptoms such as breathing problems, chest pain, discoloration of fingers and toes, dry eyes, edema, fever, hair loss, joint pain, lesions, and other rashes also may manifest. Inflammation of the kidneys, heart, lungs, blood vessels, and brain can lead to increasingly severe symptoms as the disease progresses. Patients frequently report feeling fatigue. Lupus impacts the central nervous system and the brain, causing memory problems, headaches, dizziness, behavioral changes, vision problems, and even strokes or seizures. It also can affect the blood vessels. Many patients have anemia and an increased risk of bleeding and blood clotting. Impacted blood vessels decrease blood supply to the bones, which allows tiny breaks to form, eventually leading to bone collapse. Lupus especially damages the kidneys, with kidney failure the most common cause of death among patients.

Two years after he retired, award-winning newscaster Charles Kuralt died of the disease. "Lupus runs in my family," popstar Lady Gaga revealed in 2010, shining a global spotlight on the illness.[25] Other singers, including Paula Abdul, Selena Gomez, and Seal, have publicized their struggles to raise awareness and funding for research as well.

People with lupus more frequently develop inflammation in the chest cavity lining, which can make breathing difficult. The disease's effect on blood vessels dramatically increases the chances of cardiovascular disease and heart attacks. Patients have a higher risk for infections and cancer. Doctors advise women who have lupus to delay pregnancy until they have the disease under control for at least 6 months because miscarriages are more likely during flares.

No cure exists yet, but treatments can help manage symptoms.

Multiple Sclerosis

Nerve cells in the brain and spinal cord have a fatty, protective coating called myelin, similar to insulation that protects electrical wires. An immune system malfunction that destroys that fatty coat causes multiple sclerosis (MS). If damage to the protective sheath exposes the nerve fiber, the messages that travel along those "wires" may slow or stop altogether. This process, called demyelination, causes gradual paralysis, depending on how many cells in the central nervous system sustain damage.

Low vitamin D levels, limited sunlight exposure, and smoking correlate to this disease and many other neurodegenerative illnesses. If you already suffer from another autoimmune disorder, such as thyroid disease, pernicious anemia, psoriasis, type 1 diabetes, or inflammatory bowel disease, you have a slightly higher risk of developing MS. For the most part, genetics account for only a small portion of diagnoses. Other factors, such as exposure to xenobiotics (chemicals foreign to the body, including pesticides), play a more significant role in this disease.

Multiple theories about dietary triggers have sprung up in response to the rising prevalence of autoimmune diseases in developed countries. For example, diagnoses of MS have risen in Japan, which previously had low rates of the disease. Some studies suggest that many conventionally grown coffee beans contain health-harming contaminants that not only cause short-term symptoms, such as fatigue, weakness, and brain fog (difficulty concentrating, confusion, or disorientation, but also can lead to long-term health consequences, such as cancer and neurodegenerative diseases, including MS.[26]

Growers cultivate only 3 percent of commercial coffee beans organically, meaning they treat the other 97 percent with pesticides and chemicals. Coffee crops largely come from Brazil, Colombia, Ethiopia, and other underdeveloped nations, where pesticide and chemical use often goes unregulated. Some producers use chemicals banned in America and Europe to treat their coffee plants.[27] Experts long assumed that the roasting process destroyed pesticides, but new research reveals that these chemicals can permeate the green coffee bean. As a result, roasting frequently fails to eliminate contamination, resulting in pesticide residue even in brewed coffee.

During its early stages, inflammation infiltrates the brain, optic nerve, and spinal cord, changing a person's ability to move and walk. Depending on the affected nerve tissues, signs and symptoms can vary greatly from person to person and over the course of the disease. Patients generally feel numbness or weakness in one or more limbs, which usually occurs on one side of the body at a time. Certain neck movements, particularly bending the neck forward, cause sensations of electric shock (called Lhermitte's sign). Patients can experience a lack of coordination, tremors, and a shaky gait. They can have vision issues, such as long-term double vision or blurry vision. They often experience pain when moving the eyes and can develop partial or complete loss of vision, usually in one eye at a time. They also can suffer from slurred speech, fatigue, dizziness, tingling or pain in various body parts, and sexual, bowel, or bladder dysfunction.

MS affects more than 2 million people worldwide, including Christina Applegate, Selma Blair, and Neil Cavuto. They and others have spoken about their diagnoses, making it easier for the rest of us to learn about and understand the condition. It usually strikes between the ages of 20 and 40, affecting women two to three times more than men. Recent studies indicate that the Epstein-Barr virus, which causes mononucleosis (often shortened to "mono" and sometimes called glandular fever or the kissing disease), plays an important role in its development.[28]

With MS, patients experience a cycle of remission and relapse. Remission can last months or even years. Relapses may last days or weeks, then improve partially or completely. It's a progressive disease, however, which means it gradually worsens. To date, it has no known cure, although researchers are working on identifying the triggers and biomarkers as a basis to develop prevention and additional treatment options.

Rheumatoid Arthritis

In the case of rheumatoid arthritis, the immune system attacks the joints, with peripheral damage affecting nearby bone and other related tissues. RA can run in families, so risk factors for developing the disease include genetic predisposition as well as lifestyle, specifically smoking. Ironically, alcohol consumption has an inverse association with your chances of developing RA,[29] but excessive alcohol consumption can increase the risk of psoriatic arthritis in women and of course lead to many other fatal diseases. Worldwide, more than 25 million people suffer from it, and it affects women more than twice as much as men, usually striking in middle age.

Painful and debilitating, this chronic condition causes severe difficulties for patients for the rest of their lives. Acute flares usually precede long periods of remission from the disease. In the majority of instances, the disease never stops worsening and frequently leads to almost total impairment. It can shorten a person's life expectancy by 10 years, and the number of cases rises every year.[30] Glenn Frey, Tatum O'Neal, Kathleen Turner, and Aida Turturro, among others, all shared their diagnoses with the world.

Because of the difficulty in treating this illness, the best course of action focuses on primary prevention. According to several studies, regular physical exercise reduces the likelihood of a recurrence of the condition. A dearth of major clinical studies has evaluated the impact of life habits on RA, but researchers commonly understand that eating healthy and avoiding chemical exposure, including the absorption of microplastics, can improve symptoms and severity hugely.

Anti-inflammatory medicines and immunomodulators primarily treat the disease, but successful relief generally comes from a combination of medications and behavioral modifications. While aiming for remission, it's critical to prevent further joint deterioration, control inflammation, lessen pain, and maintain muscle strength, muscle function, and quality of life.

Thyroiditis

The thyroid gland produces a variety of hormones, including thyroglobulin. It also has epithelial, or surface, cells that trigger the autoreaction in thyroiditis. In this disease, the immune system attacks thyroid cells as if they were foreign bodies, causing cell damage and cell death. When the body tries to repair the thyroid, the gland often expands, causing a decrease in thyroid hormone output. But thyroiditis, the swelling or inflammation of the thyroid gland, can lead to too much or too little production of thyroid hormones. Scientists didn't understand the condition fully until 1956, after the pioneering work of Ernest Witebsky and Noel Rose, who immunized rabbits with thyroid extracts to reproduce the disease. Deborah Doniach and Ivan Roitt later discovered thyroglobulin and thyroid antibodies.

Doctors often misdiagnose the condition because it exhibits such a wide range of symptoms potentially caused by a variety of other diseases. Developing it also depends on a number of events occurring simultaneously. It still remains unclear exactly how it arises, but genetic factors, social circumstances, infections, stress, radiation exposure, and other environmental factors can trigger onset.

You're more likely to develop thyroiditis if you already have another autoimmune disease, such as rheumatoid arthritis, type 1 diabetes, or lupus, or if you have Down syndrome or Turner syndrome. It occurs most commonly in middle-aged women, probably because of changes in immune function during pregnancy. Insufficient iodine consumption and exposure to high levels of radiation also can trigger thyroiditis.

In America, it's the most common cause of hypothyroidism (too little thyroglobulin), affecting 1 in 50 people, again mostly women. Hypothyroidism results in symptoms such as dry skin, swollen eyes, brittle hair and nails, and persistently feeling cold. Hyperthyroidism (too much thyroid hormone) affects 1 in 100 people and manifests as unwanted weight loss, high heart rate, and increased nervousness. Hashimoto's disease can cause hypothyroidism, an underactive thyroid, while Graves' disease can cause hyperthyroidism, an overactive thyroid.

Hillary Clinton, Missy Elliott, Gigi Hadid, Zoe Saldaña, Bernie Sanders, Sofia Vergara, and Oprah Winfrey all have one form or another of thyroiditis. Endocrinologists treat it with medication or thyroid replacement.

Type 1 Diabetes

In this disease, T cells target and damage the beta cells in the pancreas that produce insulin, a hormone that transports glucose, or blood sugar, from the bloodstream to cells for fuel. Doctors originally thought that only children developed this type of diabetes and that only this version of the disease required insulin treatment, so it used to be called juvenile or insulin-dependent diabetes. But we now know that adults can develop type 1 diabetes, and people with late-stage type 2 diabetes also may require insulin. Type 1 diabetes represents just 5 percent of all diabetes diagnoses.

The process can smolder in the body, unknown, for years, which means you might know someone with this kind of diabetes who hasn't been diagnosed yet. Through cell division or new growth, beta cells can reform, but over time destruction outnumbers replenishment. When the number of beta cells drops by about 80 percent, the body can't produce enough insulin, blood sugar levels increase, and clinical diabetes develops. If blood glucose levels reach unsafe levels, patients need to inject insulin to rebalance their bodies.

People with a first-degree relative (mother, father, brother, sister) who has type 1 diabetes are 15 times more likely to develop it. People with a second-degree relative (aunt, uncle, cousin) have twice the chance. Close family history poses a substantial risk factor, but roughly 85 percent of people with this disorder have no known family history of the disease. Doctors typically diagnose it in children and teenagers, and in America, white people are more likely than people of color to have type 1 diabetes. Children who develop the disease typically require insulin treatment considerably sooner and more frequently than adults with the illness—for unknown reasons.

Researchers are investigating various factors thought to activate the attack. It can result from a pancreas injury or removal, or from a viral infection, such as measles or polio. Scientists are examining cow milk proteins, vitamin D inadequacy, and omega-3 fatty acid deficiencies as possible triggers and studying the disease's relationships with viral infections, obesity, psychosocial stress, and gut microbiota. New research suggests that obesity among people with type 1 diabetes has increased faster than in the general population. Approximately half of patients with it are considered overweight or obese.[31]

Sonia Sotomayor, an associate justice of the Supreme Court of the United States, was diagnosed with type 1 diabetes at 7 years old. She's the first person serving on the court to go public with that diagnosis. She measures her blood sugar levels on a regular basis, carefully injects insulin, and always carries glucose tablets with her. She and others who manage the illness successfully do so with good dietary, environmental, and health choices.

Early genetic screening can identify who has a high risk of developing the disease. With that knowledge, physicians may be able to act sooner to shield beta cells from attack. For those who already have the condition, researchers are trying to develop drugs that can trick the immune system into not attacking or destroying the insulin-producing beta cells.

TAKE ACTION

- Have your water tested.

- If you drink coffee regularly, switch to organic.

- Know your genetic history. Find out whether any close relatives have or have had any kind of auto-immune disorder.

- Take a genetic health test to see whether you have a bio-logical predisposition to certain conditions.

- If you're at risk for developing a disorder or disease, talk to your doctor about preventive steps you can take, including important lifestyle choices.

- If you have an autoimmune condition already, tell your close family so they can make informed decisions about your health and their own.

5.

LONG HAUL: LIVING WITH VIRUSES

"It is health, which is real wealth and not pieces of gold."
—MAHATMA GANDHI

WITH AUTOIMMUNE DISEASES, YOUR BODY MISTAKENLY ATTACKS ITS OWN healthy cells, tissues, and organs. Immunodeficiencies happen when your immune system is impaired. The most well-known long-term immunodeficiency results from infection by the human immunodeficiency virus (HIV), which, when unmedicated, causes AIDS. But we live long-term with lots of viruses. Some, such as herpes type 1, rarely cause substantial problems. Some, including the varicella zoster virus, can cause difficulties, usually only later in life. The SARS coronavirus caused the deadly 2002 epidemic and 2019 pandemic, and scientists are working to understand long COVID, a condition in which the body continues responding to a coronavirus infection for many months or possibly even years.

Viruses, the most common biological entities on the planet, contain a major source of genetic diversity that, writ large, influences ecosystem dynamics. The viruses that infect us humans and cause disease constitute a tiny fraction of the whole, less than 0.1 percent. Most are harmless to you. Some even have beneficial properties, such as training your immune system. Your body conquers and eradicates some, while others remain inside you for the rest of your life. Virologists and immunologists refer to the ability of certain viruses to linger for months or years after you feel better as "persistence." Some persistent viruses can become latent, meaning they go dormant but resurface in the future, sometimes decades later. With latent viruses, there's no fond farewell.

Let's take a look at a handful of the common viruses with which we coexist.

CHICKENPOX/SHINGLES

The varicella zoster virus (VZV) causes both chickenpox and shingles. Many people caught the virus in childhood before the widespread introduction of the varicella vaccine in Asia in the 1980s and America in 1995. For those who did catch it as children, the virus remains dormant in the body for life, usually in nerve cells on either side of the spine. Later—often after acute gastric issues or as the immune system naturally declines with age—the virus can reactivate and cause shingles, a painful rash that can spread across the body. Most people who develop shingles have only one episode, but some can get it more than once. Direct contact with the fluid from rash blisters can spread VZV to people who never had chickenpox or never received the vaccine. If that happens, the recipients will develop chickenpox, not shingles, but they probably will get shingles later in life. If or when you have shingles, wear loose-fitting clothing to cover the rash completely. The virus can't spread before blisters appear or after they crust, but err on the side of caution and avoid skin-to-skin contact with others.

HERPES

Herpes simplex virus (HSV), a common infection all over the world, comes in two types. HSV-1 mostly causes infection in or around the mouth, usually in the form of cold sores, sometimes called fever blisters. But it can transfer between the mouth and genitals. HSV-2, a sexually transmitted disease (STD), causes genital herpes. It's largely asymptomatic and goes unrecognized in most healthy people, which is one reason that it spreads easily. Research into prevention and control strategies, such as vaccines and topical microbicides, is ongoing.

HIV

A classic example of a latent virus, HIV inserts its genome into the DNA of T cells and macrophages, both immune system cells. That sneaky pathway makes it invisible to the immune system. It spreads whenever carrier cells divide, a smart strategy for the virus but not great for the patient. It remains dormant for years and, if unmedicated, can trigger disease—acquired immune deficiency syndrome (AIDS)—years after the primary infection.

Until the SARS coronavirus came along, HIV was the worst pandemic most of us ever had faced. When scientists discovered AIDS in 1981, they didn't know what caused the immune disorder. Two years later, research linked it to HIV, which disrupts the immune system. If unchecked, it renders patients unable to defend themselves against bacterial, fungal, and other viral infections. Since the 1980s, HIV-AIDS research has advanced greatly. New medicines (TasP, or treatment as prevention) allow people who have the virus to live long, normal lives and help others (who use PrEP, or pre-exposure prophylaxis) to avoid infection in the first place.

LGBT+ Health

The Gay and Lesbian Medical Association held its inaugural meeting in San Francisco in June 1981, a year before I was born and in the same city where I'm writing this book. That month, the CDC reported the first cases of what later became known as AIDS. The scientific community and the world at large have endured, learned, and changed much since then. Today PrEP can prevent the transmission of HIV, TasP can subdue the virus to levels undetectable by lab tests, and people who have it can live long, healthy lives.

But stigma and ignorance continue and can result in harm both predictable and unexpected. The sexual behavior that carries the greatest risk is receptive anal sex without the use of a condom. Over the past decade, the incidence of HIV infection in America largely remained stable, but men who have sex with men (MSM) were the group most frequently diagnosed with infections. In America, HIV affects transgender people and people of color disproportionately. History points to gay male communities as the origin of the HIV-AIDS pandemic, but in some communities heterosexual people are being diagnosed with the virus at a higher rate than gay and bisexual men. In 2022, the UK Health Security Agency reported that, in England in 2020, for the first time, new diagnoses of HIV in heterosexuals (49 percent) exceeded new diagnoses in gay and bisexual men (45 percent). Viruses don't discriminate.

The wide range of complex and overlapping definitions that describe gender assignment, identity, and expression as well as sexual identity, desire, and behavior also causes difficulty. Less research has focused on LGBT+ people's risk factors for disease, such as stigma, hormone therapy, and more frequent sexual interactions that could increase potential exposure to sexually transmitted infections (STIs) or diseases. Data on transgender people proves particularly scarce. At the same time, social, medical, and legal attitudes toward issues of gender identity and sexual orientation continue to make providing appropriate healthcare for these communities an uphill battle.

Not every man who has sex with other men discloses doing so, particularly if married to a woman or otherwise not comfortable or willing to divulge his sexuality to others. As a result, it has proven difficult to avoid using self-identification as an indicator or criterion for certain vaccine rollouts. Self-identification remains too personal for general policies, and relying on it can stigmatize people who are having difficulty finding acceptance and dissuade them from taking a medication such as PrEP or getting vaccinated against a disease such as monkeypox. When the monkeypox outbreak first emerged—transmitted initially among MSM communities—I advised people in the public sphere to exercise caution when commenting about that first subset of people affected by the disease because stigma can prevent people from seeking help. I knew the virus soon would spread to the broader population, as of course it did.

Everyone can benefit from disease prevention, such as environmental regulations, water sanitation, nutrition programs, immunization initiatives, health education, nicotine cessation programs, and more, but LGBT+ people sometimes need targeted approaches with more forethought and nuance. In any medical setting, effective language and communication form the cornerstones of patient-centered care of the highest caliber. A good doctor communicates in a nonjudgmental, culturally appropriate manner, an ability crucial to any meaningful human interaction but especially so with these communities.

For LGBT+ people, improvements in governmental and medical policies, social factors, and disease prevention programs will result in the greatest improvements in immune protection and overall health. Everyone who engages in sexual activity runs the risk of acquiring STIs, but—regardless of identity, orientation, or expression—men who have sex with men and women who have sex with women both have some increased risks for particular STIs, including HIV and hepatitis. Nearly 10 percent of all new hepatitis A diagnoses involve MSM, so all MSM should receive the hepatitis A and B vaccinations.

All teenagers today must decide whether to discuss pre-exposure prophylaxis for HIV with their parents or health-care providers. Many teenagers, as they're learning about themselves, don't know what they don't know or don't feel comfortable talking to their parents about sex in general or their own sex lives in particular. If you're the parent or care-giver of a teenager, start the conversation at an appropriate age and check in with your teen periodically. Remember, diseases and infections don't discriminate, and ignorance kills. It's better to have the conversation sooner rather than too late.

HPV

A family of human papillomavirus (HPV) viruses, denoted by numbers, spreads commonly through sexual contact. Many HPV infections have no symptoms, and your body eliminates 90 percent of them after 2 years. Some infections—particularly HPV1, HPV6, and HPV11—can cause small benign tumors called papillomas or warts. Some papillomas, especially from HPV16 and HPV18, can cause genital cancers in women and men. These viruses replicate only in the basal layer of surface tissues, such as the skin or mucosal epithelium of the genitals, anus, mouth, or airways. HPV1 infects the soles of the feet, while HPV2 affects the palms of the hands. To date, three HPV vaccines are available (only one in America) to protect the body from cancer caused by

HPV, but they're age specific: at around 11 or 12 or before 27 years old.

SARS CORONAVIRUS

Named for their crown-like molecular structure, coronaviruses are a family of RNA viruses that infect various animals. The common cold, as we know it, results from four coronaviruses. SARS-CoV-1 caused the 2002 SARS pandemic, and SARS-CoV-2 caused COVID-19. As we all have seen recently, the virus can provoke vastly different outcomes in different people, and some of that comes down to patients' immune systems.

A strong immune system isn't always a good thing. In certain conditions, it can be a liability. The 1918 influenza pandemic and the 2019 coronavirus pandemic proved so lethal for some otherwise healthy people for precisely this reason. Some patients improved, then declined rapidly. Some survivors took months to recover, and others developed long-term immune challenges. An *optimized* immune system offers the best defense now and in the future because it arms your body with powerful tools to defeat infections and diseases that will try to invade.

When faced with viral threats, your body responds with immune cells and inflammatory cells. Inflammation, as we've seen, is a biological response of the immune system that bacteria, food, toxins, synthetic materials, viruses, and other factors can trigger. Every major organ and various systems in the body may experience severe or chronic inflammation as a result of immune responses. The cell damage that they sustain, in turn, can activate even more inflammatory reactions. When that mechanism goes unchecked, it can trigger a systemic, life-threatening response called a cytokine storm. If the body is too weak to counter or balance its own cytokine storm, it shuts down and the patient dies.

Cytokine Storms

It's the most terrifying clinical scenario for any doctor to encounter. Everything goes wrong simultaneously. When the body can't fend off a cytokine storm in one place, the inflammatory response spreads to other organs, resulting in cytokine storm syndrome (CSS). Cytokines, as we saw in Chapter 1, perform many functions. They help develop antibodies, recruit other immune cells, prompt blood to clot more easily, and lessen the body's inflammatory response. That's right, some cytokines cause inflammation and others reduce it. In CSS, the inflammatory ones outnumber their anti-inflammatory siblings and "storm" your body. Various autoimmune disorders, cancers, pathogens, and even therapies can cause this hyperactivation.

An alarming number of CSS patients wind up in multiorgan system failure, which is the medical phrase for being on the verge

Cytokine Storm

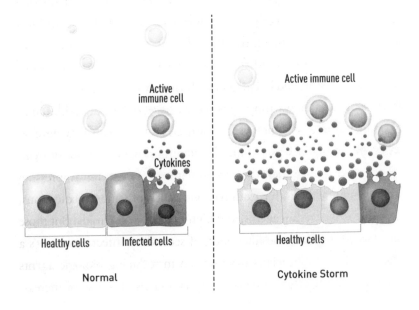

Normal — Healthy cells · Infected cells · Active immune cell · Cytokines

Cytokine Storm — Active immune cell · Healthy cells

of death. If you've seen someone having a panic attack, you know how much effort it can take for someone to calm down. Imagine a body-wide panic attack where none of the systems is listening. The phenomenon first appeared in medical literature in 1952, but only a handful of publications touched on it until the mid-1970s. Different investigators in different fields have studied it, which has resulted unhelpfully in different names with different descriptions of it. Because it affects different parts of the body, it calls for the attention of different clinicians, including infectious disease specialists and oncologists. But physicians are struggling to agree on diagnostic criteria. The earlier that doctors recognize, diagnose, and treat CSS, the better the outcome. Unfortunately, because it has so many triggers and happens everywhere all at once, physicians frequently can misdiagnose or not even recognize it until too late in the process, making treatment ineffective.

But as with so many other areas of life, COVID-19 changed that, too. The rise in CSS cases that the disease caused has created renewed interest in this disorder. Before COVID, one of the most common triggers for CSS was influenza. Medical historians consider CSS largely responsible for many of the 50 million deaths worldwide during the 1918 flu pandemic. For reasons that we still don't understand fully, the SARS coronavirus that causes COVID-19 more likely triggers CSS than other viruses.[32]

One of the first warning signs is early onset of fever. In addition to the initial infection, if not caught early enough, patients may develop CSS and bacterial sepsis, a life-threatening situation. Primary treatments for CSS dampen the inflammatory response by suppressing the immune system, for example, with chemotherapy medications, lymphocyte-targeting agents, and high-dose corticosteroids. But those approaches increase the likelihood of secondary infections, so it's a delicate dance. Clinicians have started introducing biologic agents that specifically target inflammatory cytokines. The rise of increasingly personalized medicine, thanks to continued pharmaceutical advancement, may drastically reduce the number of deaths from CSS.

Long COVID

Those who survive viral infections and possible cytokine storms aren't always in the clear, however. Some people experience symptoms for a couple of days, while others still have symptoms weeks later. In the worst cases, symptoms linger for months and even years. Early studies in Europe found that 87 percent of patients discharged from the hospital had persistent symptoms.[33] Even patients with mild symptoms, who never needed hospitalization, can suffer from post-COVID conditions. Dubbed long COVID, this post-acute sequelae of COVID-19 (PASC) poses multiple challenges to our health, society, and future. The CDC uses PASC as an umbrella term for "new, returning, or ongoing health problems" experienced by people 4 weeks or more after a SARS coronavirus infection.

As an advisor to legislators and a member of Covid Act Now—a not-for-profit organization designing and evaluating data-driven epidemiological models of the pandemic that the White House presented in press briefings—I have seen PASC strike firsthand. Before the pandemic, Gilberto Lopes, one of my friends and colleagues, a world-renowned lung cancer specialist, and a medical oncologist, could run 5 kilometers in fewer than 30 minutes. During the early months of the pandemic, he contracted the virus.

His infection began mildly, with a runny nose and a scratchy throat, before breaking into a fever. For the next 10 days, his temperature reached 102.8°F, which he alleviated temporarily with a combination of anti-inflammatories and rest. Later, even when resting, he experienced shortness of breath. His doctor prescribed dexamethasone, a powerful corticosteroid, but it didn't allay the inflammatory response. As Lopes's oxygen levels declined, his trips to the emergency room became more frequent, until ultimately the hospital admitted him. When he checked in, he was suffering from chronic headaches, mental fog, delirium, and hallucinations

After receiving remdesivir, a powerful antiviral medication, and more powerful anti-inflammatories, he began to feel better. He was one of the lucky ones who didn't have to go on a ventilator, his greatest fear. But during his ordeal, he lost 14 pounds. Long after the hospital discharged him, he has had trouble gaining that weight back and regaining his stamina. In the middle of an easy run, he still has to stop to catch his breath, and he continues to deal with brain fog. His case and millions more like it offer empirical proof that you don't have to be unhealthy or have the most severe form of COVID to have long-lasting symptoms.

Millions of people have recovered from the illness, but its symptoms can linger because the virus can harm the lungs, heart, and brain, increasing the likelihood of long-term health issues. Researchers continue working to understand the underlying mechanisms more fully, but they believe PASC has a few potential causes: residual organ damage from the body's own immune response, remnants of the virus lingering in one or more organs, and an overly active immune response in some people. Every day, new research adds another piece to the puzzle, but the picture remains far from complete. As long as people keep catching this brutal virus, which already has killed more than 6 million people worldwide, we will continue to see more long COVID cases emerge.

Risk Factors

Chronic illness and long COVID share many common risk factors and antecedents, such as advanced age, diabetes, smoking, malnutrition or obesity, immunosuppression, and hypertension. Other factors also complicate the issue: the time between onset of acute and chronic symptoms; a lack of understanding of post-COVID and post-ICU pathology, which sometimes leads to a failure to connect the dots; and the chicken-and-egg question of whether critical illness causes post-COVID illnesses or preexisting conditions push patients with low resiliency past the tipping point. Here are four known risk factors for developing COVID-19 and, by extension, long COVID:

1. **Age.** Elderly people have a higher risk of contracting infectious diseases because over time your immune system naturally declines. Data sets from America, Canada, China, Italy, Japan, Singapore, and South Korea reveal an age-dependent disparity in COVID susceptibility. Preexisting conditions, or comorbidities, are more common in older populations. They are more likely to have weakened immune defenses as well as higher inflammatory responses, which results in greater tissue damage from infections. Elderly people have higher levels of proinflammatory cytokines, which create cytokine storms.

2. **Sex.** According to pandemic reports from around the world, males make up the vast majority of COVID patients.[34] Females generally are more resistant to infections than males. Different hormone effects in inflammatory processes, different levels of particular cell receptors and molecules, and lifestyle differences, such as smoking and drinking, may predispose males to COVID infection as well.

3. **Race and ethnicity.** Social, racial, and ethnic disparities heavily influence the outcomes of COVID patients. According to a systemic analysis of studies conducted in the United Sates, populations of color had higher rates of infection and mortality than Caucasian populations, while Asian populations had similar rates of infections,

hospitalizations, and deaths.[35] According to the COVID-19 Cardiovascular Disease Registry study from the American Heart Association (AHA), Hispanic and Black patients disproportionately accounted for more than half of all hospitalizations and more than half of all in-hospital deaths.[36]

4. **Health problems.** Patients with underlying conditions are more vulnerable to the SARS coronavirus because their preexisting diseases have weakened their immune systems, predisposing them to infection. The most common comorbidities reported in American COVID patients were hypertension, diabetes, cardiovascular disease, and chronic kidney disease.[37]

More research will identify other potential risk factors and preventive measures, clarify the underlying mechanisms of the body's response to infection, and help develop new treatments. But this won't be the last virus to cause long-term illness, which is why having an optimized immune system is so vital.

Symptoms

The SARS coronavirus can affect multiple organs in the body. As a result, long COVID leads to a variety of symptoms, including respiratory, neurological, cardiac, and psychological issues. These are some of the long-term signs and symptoms of long COVID:

- fatigue
- headache
- breathing problems
- chest pain or discomfort
- cough
- decline or loss of sense of smell and/or taste
- muscle pain, aches, or weakness
- joint pain

- throat irritation
- memory loss
- brain fog
- dizziness
- low-grade, sporadic fever
- heart palpitations or irregular heartbeats
- anxiety
- depression
- post-traumatic stress disorder (PTSD)
- insomnia
- earache, hearing loss, and/or tinnitus (ringing in the ears)
- rashes
- nausea, abdominal pain, and/or diarrhea
- appetite decrease
- hair loss

Some people may have only one or two of these symptoms, while others might develop more. Symptoms differ greatly from person to person. To date, no single test can diagnose long COVID. Doctors identify it in part by looking at your COVID history and ruling out other possibilities. Your doctor will ask whether you ever tested positive for COVID, when symptoms first appeared, and what symptoms you've had since the infection. Your doctor will inquire about underlying medical issues and test your blood pressure, heart rate, oxygen levels, and breathing.

Respiratory symptoms might call for a chest X-ray. An electro-cardiogram (ECG or EKG) painlessly measures heart activity for patients with cardiac symptoms. Blood work may offer insights as well. Physical tests include a 6-minute walking test and a test in which you must sit in and stand up from a chair five times. Depending on your symptoms, you might undergo cognitive or psychological testing, which could consist of a screening questionnaire and/or short tests to evaluate memory, language ability, reasoning, and other cognitive skills. For some long-haulers, symptoms resolve within 3 months of the initial infection. Other patients may experience symptoms for much longer.

Treatment

Vaccination cuts your risk of developing long COVID in half.[38] It's the most critical strategy for prevention and mitigation. The mRNA COVID vaccines will help you avoid severe disease and death.

VACCINES

Vaccines come in several different types. Live, attenuated vaccines contain a weakened version of a virus or bacteria that's unable to cause damage to your system. They're the closest thing to the real deal and make good teachers for your immune system. Inactivated vaccines, such as the polio inoculation, contain an inactivated or dead germ. The COVID vaccine is an mRNA vaccine, which means it doesn't contain any piece of the microbe that it fights. mRNA vaccines use lab-made messenger RNA to tell your body how to make a protein needed to fight an infection.

Many clinical trials for various COVID vaccine candidates are ongoing. These include attenuated vaccines, inactivated vaccines, mRNA vaccines, vector-based vaccines, subunit vaccines, and DNA vaccines. In a recent pilot study, people with a prior COVID infection produced much higher levels of antibodies after a single dose of the Pfizer vaccine, compared to those without prior infection, indicating that vaccination boosts the immune system's memory and can help prevent reinfections.[39] Further data on dosage, timing, overall efficacy, performance against variants, and duration of protection will help medical officials improve their approaches to fighting the virus and its consequences.

You also can mitigate your risk of getting COVID or long COVID by adopting a healthy lifestyle and eating nutritious foods. Vitamins (specifically C and D) and minerals, proteins, dietary fiber, short-chain fatty acids, and omega-3 polyunsaturated fatty acids may help during an infection and improve a prognosis. Vitamin D in particular plays an important role in the immune system. A recent study found that patients with severe COVID had lower levels of 25-OH vitamin D in their blood than people with mild cases as well as a noninfected control group.[40] So vitamin D deficiency may put you at greater risk of critical illness. Vitamin C decreases inflammatory cytokines and increases anti-inflammatory cytokines.

Depending on type and severity, patients with multiple symptoms may need attention from specialists in cardiology, pulmonology, neurology, otolaryngology, psychiatry, rehabilitation, and other fields. No one medication or therapy can treat long COVID. Some symptom-specific, medically supervised treatments include:

- **Fatigue.** Learn more about the four Ps: pacing, planning, prioritizing, and positioning. Consider a special stretching, strengthening, or aerobic exercise program. If exercise aggravates your symptoms, stop or reduce the activity's intensity or duration.
- **Lungs.** Breathing exercises, supplemental oxygen, and pulmonary rehabilitation can help. A pulse oximeter can monitor your oxygen saturation levels. If your blood oxygen saturation drops below 92 percent, seek medical help.
- **Heart.** Medications and cardiac rehabilitation can alleviate certain symptoms.
- **Nervous system.** Exercise and other physical activity may help with cognitive symptoms, such as memory loss or

brain fog. Memory exercises and aids, including calendars and planners, can help with memory impairment.

- **Mind.** Counseling, support groups, and medications commonly treat depression, anxiety, and other psychiatric conditions.

- **Odor and taste.** Topical corticosteroids can help improve a lost or diminished sense of smell or taste. In olfactory training, patients sniff various odors on a regular basis, usually for several weeks.

TAKE ACTION

- Gather your vaccination records and make sure all your vaccines are up to date.

- If you had chickenpox as a child, plan to get the shingles vaccine. If you've had shingles, also get the vaccine.

- If you have shingles, wear loose-fitting clothes that completely cover the rash.

- If you're sexually active, get regular HIV tests and talk to your healthcare provider about PrEP or TasP.

- If you have a child younger than age 10, talk to your pediatrician about HPV vaccination. If you're not yet 27 years old, talk to your doctor about catch-up vaccination.

- The next time you get sick, supplement with vitamins C and D to bolster your immune system.

- Whenever you become eligible for COVID vaccines or boosters, get them. Mix manufacturers for maximum coverage.

- If you have two or more symptoms of long COVID, talk to your doctor about treatment options.

PART TWO

YOUR HEALTHIER FUTURE

6.

INFORMATION IS POWER

"The only reason for time is so that everything doesn't happen at once."

—Albert Einstein

ONE OF THE BEST TOOLS IN YOUR QUEST TO OPTIMIZE YOUR IMMUNE SYSTEM is information. The more you know about your body, how it works, what best suits it, and which tweaks will result in better health, the easier it becomes to create a whole-body plan for you to live a healthier, longer life. In Part One, we looked at genetic testing, but other tests can reveal how your body is working, enabling you to create healthier habits.

CHRONOBIOLOGY

Natural rhythms, such as light, seasons, sounds, and vibrations, affect all living organisms. Chronobiology, the study of those rhythms, examines, for example, why birds migrate, why trees drop their leaves in the fall, and why you fall asleep at night and wake up in the morning. Deep within your body, biological timers control the fundamental rhythms of your life. Understanding how natural rhythms impact your health can help you improve your life by

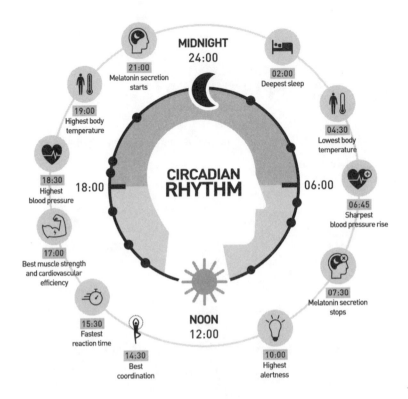

tweaking daily habits, such as the best time to eat a meal or take a medication, for example.

For centuries, scientists noticed that plants and animals followed rhythms and patterns—sleeping at night, active by day, for instance—but no one studied the phenomena carefully until the 18th century. Astronomer Jean-Jacques d'Ortous de Mairan observed a mimosa plant's daily leaf movements, opening in the morning and closing at night, regardless of whether the plant stood in sunlight or darkness. He partnered with another scientist, botanist Jean Marchant, to write and present a paper. Other scientists added to their research and tested the theory further by putting the plant in various controlled settings, including reversing the light and dark times. The results remained the same: The plant returned to its natural, endogenous (internal) rhythm of opening its leaves in the morning and closing them at night. This observation revealed that the rhythms resulted not from external stimuli. We humans like to think that we stand apart from all the other life forms, but the opposite holds true.

You result from eons of evolution and connect to every part of the earth. The nitrogen in your DNA, the calcium in your teeth, and the iron in your blood all trace back millions of years to thousands of collapsing stars. It's not science fiction; it's science. While your telomeres track your biological age, an internal clock regulates other systems, including sleep, nutrition, physical activity, and even sex.

FLOWER TIME

Plants' chronobiologies are so predictable that Swedish naturalist Carl Linnaeus designed a flower clock in 1751. He arranged certain flowering plants in a circular pattern, using the points in the day that the flowers opened to mark time. The hawk's-beard plant, for instance, opens its flowers at 6:30 a.m., while the hawkbit plant does so at 7 a.m.

Well-known scientists, including Georg Lichtenberg, Christoph Hufeland, Carl Linnaeus, and Charles Darwin, observed and reported these rhythmic phenomena. But chronobiology research didn't really get underway and expand into human applications until the 20th century. Today, a thorough understanding of these patterns proves critical in the prevention and treatment of diseases as well as the healing process.

Biorhythms

In the 1950s, Franz Halberg was testing eosinophil levels in mouse blood and realized that the numbers differed, depending on time of day. He also noted that the phenomenon extended to other parts of the mice. Glycogen levels in their livers and the total number of cells dividing also varied greatly throughout the day. After collecting the data and examining the patterns as a function of time, he noticed predictable 24-hour cycles. He converted the data to a graph and saw a pattern of peaks and valleys, day after day. "Circa" (around) every 24 hours, or day (*dies* in Latin), the patterns recurred, and so they became known as circadian rhythms.

Your body has four essential biorhythms, in order of length: ultradian (fewer than 24 hours), diurnal (night and day), circadian (24 hours), and infradian (more than 24 hours). Your body behaves organically, meaning that it consumes organic materials and functions in organic cycles. It seeks to follow the same patterns, day after day. It "turns on" when you wake and reboots when you go to sleep, much like a computer. It consistently follows or tries to follow these rhythms, which is why it's so crucial to maintain healthy routines.

Changing, interrupting, or stopping your bio clock can harm your health, moods, and mental activity. Jet lag, for instance, results from traveling swiftly to a different time zone, particularly one several or more hours from your own. Your circadian rhythm synchs to your time zone, so the differences in daylight—including the sun rising and setting at different times—confuses your body. Most people experience it as temporary fatigue and general malaise, possibly with some dizziness or nausea, but some sufferers, particularly when traveling to different hemispheres, develop brain fog and need several days to adjust.

HOW TO MINIMIZE JET LAG

In the days prior to departure, gradually adjust your schedule to the new time zone. Get plenty of rest before you leave. No all-nighters doing laundry and packing. Adjust to the new schedule by taking melatonin an hour or so before it's time to sleep in the destination time zone.

Use a soundscape app that triggers sleepiness, such as the Endel app, or a device that generates electromagnetic brain waves related to sleep, such as NeoRhythm. Drink lots of water before, during, and after travel.

Your biological clock not only influences your organs and cells, but it also regulates what are called clock-controlled genes. Over the course of a 24-hour period, approximately 20 percent of your genes turn on and off to perform different bodily functions. Just as with de Mairan's mimosa plants, your internal clock, which your hypothalamus ultimately controls, doesn't require external signals to function. That means that your body knows, under normal circumstances, when it should sleep and when it should wake up in every 24-hour period. But your environment plays a role, too.[41] Your age, gender, and even the time of year all affect how your body responds to exterior influences on your circadian rhythm. Light, temperature, and food—collectively *zeitgebers,* German for "time donors"—affect it, too. They can change your sleep, hormones, mental stamina, and even eating patterns.

People who work nights, for instance, disrupt their circadian rhythms, which can cause dire health consequences. Circadian biorhythms affect body temperature, which drops by approximately

1°C in the dark; sodium and potassium excretion through the urine; and different hormones, including melatonin, which varies according to the light-dark cycle of the day; growth hormone, which reaches maximum levels in the early morning; and cortisol, which peaks in the morning when you wake. During the first half of the day, your digestive system secretes more enzymes than before bed. That secretion optimizes digestion all day, and for the same reason, eating late at night can give you indigestion. Scientists can measure all of these levels.

Melatonin is one of the most effective antioxidants. Significantly reducing it can cause oxidative distress and increased inflammation. Since Halberg's discovery, other scientists have taken circadian maps of various bodily activities—resistance to stimuli, cell divisions in different organs and tissues, liver function—and applied that knowledge to treating cancer and other diseases. From these discoveries, the new fields of chronopharmacology and chronotherapy have risen. At different times of the day, your body resists or yields to different stimuli, which has advanced our understanding of how circadian rhythms affect medications. Future studies probably will find a link between sleep deficiencies and an increased risk of developing cancer and other conditions stemming from high levels of proinflammatory cytokines.

Light Exposure and Sleep Disruption

By design, your circadian clock reacts well to sunlight. Studies show that increased exposure to sunlight can improve your sleep, energy levels, and health.[43] For people with jet lag, other studies have demonstrated that phased exposure to natural light gradually changes the biological clock until it aligns with the clock on the wall.[44]

Some people wake up ready to take on the world; others feel groggy and take a long time to feel awake after rising. A former colleague used to say that her brain didn't get going until she had at least one cup of coffee. Caffeine stimulated her system to overcome her sleep inertia. A temporary, sleep-related lack of cognitive performance and awareness, sleep inertia makes it hard for many people to wake in the morning. It usually passes in half an hour or less, but for some unlucky people that lingering feeling of drowsiness can last for up to 4 hours.

The pattern of your sleep cycles can impact your tendency to experience sleep inertia. Early birds get their deepest sleep a few hours before the sun rises, so they wake in a light-sleep state. I'm one of those people. I naturally wake before dawn. Night owls who work or live on regular human time have it the worst, though, because they regularly have to interrupt a deep-sleep state to realign themselves with the rest of the world. Jarring your body from deep sleep makes it harder to get back to normal, which is why night owls often start their days feeling groggy. It's also why you should never hit snooze on a wake-up alarm. When it goes off, get up and stay up. Even better, track your sleep needs

TIMING MEDICATIONS

For approximately 30 percent of medications, *when* is just as important as how much. Enzymes controlling cholesterol production are most active at night, so taking a drug such as Lipitor in the evening makes more sense. The same rationale applies to blood pressure. Taking medication for high blood pressure at night capitalizes on the body's natural production rhythm. This strategy has helped reduce the incidence of nighttime heart attacks by 45 percent.[42]

and use an alarm to remind yourself to go to bed, instead of one to wake you.

Alcohol and stimulants such as caffeine also can cause sleep inertia because they disrupt your natural sleep cycles. Long naps can cause problems, too. Limit naps to no more than 30 minutes. Sleeping longer than that will pull you into a deep sleep cycle, which can make you feel more tired. If sleep inertia regularly impairs your quality of life, talk to your healthcare provider about what else you can do to improve your quality of sleep.

One of the most disruptive environmental factors, blue light also can push your body's cycles forward or backward. Some poultry farmers modify the biology of their birds by exposing them to artificial lights on a regular basis. Blue light confuses and stresses the body, so it's important to wear an eye mask when going to sleep. Blue light exposure can result in melatonin deficiency and sleep deprivation, which, in turn, reduce your body's immune response and the nightly release of cortisol, which increases your risk for insulin resistance, obesity, and type 2 diabetes.

BLUE LIGHT WEIGHT GAIN

If, at night, you watch a lot of TV or stare at your phone, that blue light is sending the wrong signals to your brain. It can lead to weight gain because, while you're sleeping, you aren't producing as much cortisol, which regulates your metabolism. For a healthier weight and a better night's sleep, no electronics while in bed and keep your sleeping space dark. If you absolutely can't break the habit, apply an anti–blue light or nighttime filter to any screen you use after sunset.

Sleep duration also alters your biological clock, eating habits, and weight. Too little sleep interferes with your production of ghrelin, the hormone responsible for hunger, and leptin, the hormone linked to feeling full. These hormones "alert" your brain when to eat and when to stop, but you still have agency in the situation. If your ghrelin is running high and leptin low, you may wake hungry and craving carbohydrates, but you shouldn't eat a whole loaf of bread. When your body tells you it's hungry, you choose how to fuel it.

In 1969, only 15 percent of Americans slept fewer than 7 hours a night. Today, almost half do.[45] For most people, that's the magic number. Fewer than 7 hours risks all the negative outcomes above. More than 7 hours gives your body enough time to reset. That threefold increase in sleep deficits in recent decades has contributed to the obesity epidemic. Unfortunately, obesity impairs the immune system, which in turn opens the door to infections and disease. A few nights of bad sleep won't destroy your overall health, but a chronic pattern of poor sleep can lead to increased calorie intake, weight gain, obesity, type 2 diabetes, and other problems. Think of a road with ruts carved over centuries by countless wheels. If one vehicle goes slightly east, it won't change the ruts. If several thousand cars drive east, they'll form a new rut that will take future drivers to a different destination.

For research, Stefania Follini spent 4 months in a cave so dark she never saw the sun or the moon. The absence of light disoriented her mentally and physically. She lost track of time, thinking that only 2 months had passed when 4 had elapsed. Her menstrual cycles stopped, and she lost 17 pounds. With no visuals to influence her circadian rhythm, her sleep varied from a handful of hours to a whopping 35.[46]

Lunar Living

Recent scientific research acknowledges that, while the moon can't predict your future or trigger werewolf transformations, lunar cycles do affect human biology by influencing menstrual and sleep cycles.[47]

An analysis of sleep cycles in rural and urban indigenous Argentinians as well as urban American university students indicated that, on the nights leading to a full moon, when more and more moonlight fills the night sky, people fall asleep later and sleep less.[48] The findings imply that, independent of ethnic or cultural differences, sleep cycles sync with the moon—even in areas where light pollution outshines moonlight.

Most women's menstrual cycles synchronize at regular intervals with the synodic month, or a complete moon cycle (new moon to full moon). The periods of women aged 35 and younger synchronize with the full or new moon 23.6 percent of the time. Surprisingly, only 9.5 percent of women over age 35 demonstrate that synchronicity. Menstrual cycles also coincide with the tropical month—the 27.32 days it takes the moon to pass twice through the same point in its orbit—13.1 percent of the time in women 35 or younger and 17.7 percent of the time in women older than 35, which implies that changes in the moon's gravitational pull also affect menstruation.[49]

So it turns out that astrologers may have been right all along. The movement of celestial bodies does influence our lives, including fertility and sleep.

Sound Therapy

Noise can exacerbate or alleviate stress, help or hinder learning and memory, and aid or interrupt sleep. I have been working with Endel, an app that integrates sound into daily activities. The app creates real-time, personalized soundscapes based on chronobiology research and cutting-edge acoustic technology to help with focus, relaxation, and sleep. When using the app with noise-canceling headphones for work-related tasks, my productivity improves dramatically. Many audio-streaming services offer curated playlists designed to increase your focus during specific time intervals.

In several studies, natural sounds such as white noise and classical music also increased focus and improved learning outcomes. A great nonpharmaceutical tool, soundscapes like those can help you sleep, relax, or focus. On the other hand, listening to music with lyrics while reading or working can reduce concentration and cognitive performance.

CHRONONUTRITION

The relationships among mealtimes, metabolism, physiology, and the body's internal clock collectively constitute the field of chrononutrition. It aims to create eating habits in harmony with biorhythms, maximize energy levels, and improve health. Three biorhythms relate to chrononutrition: ultradian (fewer than 24 hours, such as heart rate); circadian (24 hours); and infradian (more than 24 hours, such as a menstrual cycle). As we have seen, metabolism, digestion, and hormone secretion all tie to circadian rhythms, which means there may be better and worse times to eat.

Certain digestive functions have a daily regularity. Your stomach empties most quickly in the morning. Beta cells, which make insulin, function 15 percent faster in the morning. Insulin sensitivity decreases through the day. Eating when your insulin sensitivity runs low (at night) can lead to insulin resistance, reduced energy, and obesity. Thermogenesis, the energy your body needs to digest and absorb your food, is 44 percent lower in the evening than in the morning. You are more likely to experience blood sugar spikes in the evening, even if your 3-month A1C levels (glucose-linked hemoglobin) are consistent. Chronodisruption—going to sleep late at night, blue-light exposure after dark—affects your appetite hormones and food cravings.

The connection between circadian rhythms and chrononutrition points to times to eat and times to avoid eating. Analyzing my glucose levels, biological age, and overall health revealed that my chronobiological schedule functions best when I hydrate abundantly all day but eat only once a day. So I shifted to one meal per day—with some exceptions. My mental stamina improved tremendously, and I feel 25 years old.

Published in 2019 in the *British Medical Journal*, a collection of 13 studies on breakfast and weight loss found that people who eat breakfast consume more calories and weigh more than those who skip breakfast.[50] Multiple studies have demonstrated that skipping breakfast helps with weight loss and metabolic disorders. Your body doesn't need food first thing in the morning because hormones give you enough energy to jump-start your day. Nor is your body ready to break down all those fats and carbs as soon as you wake up. Delaying or skipping breakfast entirely cuts unnecessary intake and decreases the consumption of unhealthy foods, such as ultraprocessed cereals and other sugary foods. Morning fasting also correlates to lower incidence of heart disease, high blood pressure, and high cholesterol.[51]

Glucose Monitoring

What's your blood-glucose level right now? What happens in your body after you eat a bagel? Is the impact different if you eat an apple or a handful of carrots?

Blood sugar, or blood glucose, carries energy to your cells. When your levels run low (hypoglycemia), you can feel fatigued and weak and experience headaches and dizziness. Blood sugar levels that run high (hyperglycemia) disrupt your insulin balance, which can lead to all kinds of medical problems, including diabetes, kidney disease, heart attacks, and strokes. Many factors, including activity levels and your overall lifestyle, can affect blood sugar. Knowing your levels can help you find ideal targets for energy efficiency in your body.

January AI offers a special metabolic health program called the Season of Me, a 90-day guided plan to maximize health through small, easy steps such as monitoring blood glucose throughout the day. A device and app work together to reveal the glycemic load of foods and how they impact glucose, tracked using heart rate and continuous glucose monitors (CGM). Continuous monitoring reduces hypoglycemia and hyperglycemia in people with insulin-treated diabetes, but its value for people with prediabetes and non-insulin-treated type 2 diabetes remains unclear to scientists. I don't have any of those conditions, but I found the program beneficial because it helped me understand how my body reacts to different food groups.

Traditional fingerstick tests record one blood-glucose level at a single point in time. It's like reading only one page of a book. Additional fingerstick checks provide more snapshots of your blood sugars. A great tool for people with diabetes, a CGM—used only under the care of a physician—goes beneath the surface of your skin and constantly reads your glucose levels. The results transmit to a wearable device or smartphone. By seeing how your body reacts to a bagel or a carrot, you can make better decisions about your food choices. The Season of Me program showed me that some of the foods I used to eat on a daily basis caused my blood sugar to spike. This allowed me to make simple but effective changes for my health.

Diabetes affects everyone differently. One food or activity affects one person's glucose levels in a different way from another person. All of which can make managing diabetes difficult, even when following all the recommended procedures. Your body behaves according to the instructions you give it, but sometimes it still reacts unpredictably. That's why it's so important to gather as much information about it as possible so you can have better conversations about your health with your doctors—and of course so you can live better.

Food Allergies

Sensitivities and allergies to food constitute two distinct illnesses that necessitate different sets of diagnostic tests. Food intolerance may cause bothersome symptoms, such as stomach rumbling, discomfort, or diarrhea. A true allergy may cause life-threatening symptoms.

In an allergic reaction, your immune system overreacts to a perceived intruder by sending antibodies called immunoglobulin E (IgE) to attack it. Symptoms from a food allergy usually appear within minutes of eating and can affect any body system, including the skin, mouth, gastrointestinal system, respiratory system, and cardiovascular system. The reaction can range from a mild rash or oral swelling to difficulty breathing or anaphylaxis, a potentially life-threatening inflammatory response that manifests rapidly and often affects two or more organ systems at once. Anaphylaxis often requires an immediate injection of epinephrine.

In America, 42.3 percent of children with a food allergy have reported having a severe food-allergic reaction. One of every five children with a food allergy has reported visiting an emergency department for an allergic reaction in the previous year. Severity varies according to age and allergen. According to the American Academy of Pediatrics, most of the severe reactions and emergency room visits result from exposure to peanuts and tree nuts or seeds.[52]

Allergic Reaction

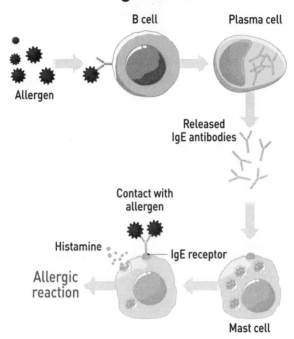

Peanut Problems and Protocols

Lectins, phytoestrogens, and aflatoxins—known allergens for large portions of the population—exist in many common foods.[53] Some legumes have a lot of lectins. Others, such as soybeans, contain a lot of phytoestrogens. Peanuts have lots of aflatoxins. Isoflavones are estrogen-like chemicals found in foods rich in soy. Research shows that these substances can boost cancer cell growth, impair female fertility, and disrupt thyroid function. Lectins, found in legumes, dairy, and nightshade plants, can lead to intestinal diseases in some people.[54] As allergens, their toxic capacity can induce a variety of health issues ranging from bloating and nausea to vomiting and loose stools, among other problems.

Peanuts, in particular, prove problematic. In addition to having the potential to kill someone allergic to them, peanuts contain a lot of saturated fat, which can lead to heart problems if you eat them regularly. Peanuts also have a high concentration of phosphorus, which can interfere with your body's ability to absorb other minerals, such as zinc and iron. After researching their impact on human health, I gave up eating them entirely. If you're sensitive to them, you should, too.

But clinical trials on peanut desensitization have yielded promising results, particularly for children younger than age 4.[55] An examination of open-label trials published between 2009 and 2010 revealed substantial rates of desensitization, ranging from 64 to 93 percent depending on criteria, method, and outcomes. This oral immunotherapy method (OIT) essentially gives the allergic person an increasing amount of that allergen to raise the threshold before triggering a reaction. In an allergist's office or clinical research setting, the dose gradually increases over a period of months, until the sensitivity level decreases to the point where inadvertent consumption won't result in anaphylactic shock. OIT has desensitized 60 to 80 percent of patients with peanut, egg, and milk sensitivities.[56] It can't eliminate an allergy, but it can give people with serious food allergies more freedom.

FAMILY ALLERGIES

Allergies frequently come in groups. If you're sensitive to latex, you also might be allergic to apples, apricots, or avocados. If you're allergic to strawberries, you're probably also allergic to celery, kiwifruit, melons, nectarines, papayas, and wheat. Food sensitivities and intolerances are extremely common. Experts believe that somewhere between 2 and 20 percent of the world's population has some kind of food intolerance.

The FDA recently approved peanut allergen powder (brand name Palforzia) as the first drug for treating peanut allergies in children.[57] Kids between ages 4 and 17 with a proven peanut allergy can get this medication to help prevent responses such as anaphylaxis.

Food Allergy Testing

Many people live their whole lives with bloating and gastrointestinal issues, not realizing those side effects come from consuming allergens. In my career, I've seen more patients with food allergies than I can count. So how do you know if you have a food allergy?

The marketplace has lots of at-home tests. Everlywell and Viome are two of the most dependable. Neither needs a doctor's order, and you can do either at home. Viome combines data from a microbiome test with a metabolic test to determine how your body and the flora in your digestive system interact with distinct foods. From there, you receive a customized plan to help you stay balanced and run at your performance peak without food sensitivities slowing you down.

More tests are coming, but the absolute best way to know is to visit an allergist. An allergist typically will use multiple forms of analysis—usually medical history, symptom reporting, skin prick tests, and IgE testing—to make a diagnosis. An elimination diet followed by oral challenge testing often joins blood or skin tests to determine a food allergy. At-home tests lack this rigorous approach, so keep your healthcare provider informed.

Each food receives a rating on a class scale from 0 to 3:

- Class 0, normal reactivity
- Class 1, minimal reactivity
- Class 2, some reactivity
- Class 3, high reactivity

A higher reactivity level can indicate a food might be triggering symptoms, making it an ideal candidate for testing in an elimination diet and add-back challenge.

Heavy Metals

As you'll recall from the periodic table of elements, metals are shiny, usually malleable, and conduct heat and electricity. Heavy metals, as the name indicates, have high densities. They also have high toxicity levels in humans. You can breathe them in, ingest them, or absorb them through your skin. If too many metals enter your body, you run the risk for heavy metal poisoning, which can cause cognitive problems, behavioral abnormalities, and organ damage. The type and amount of metal determine symptoms and their impact. You probably encounter the following three common heavy metals every day.

Mercury

Released into the air through emissions from power plants and burning fossil fuels, mercury settles on lakes and oceans, where fish and shellfish absorb it. When you eat mercury-tainted fish or shellfish, you ingest this poisonous metal. A study from the Biodiversity Research Institute found that 84 percent of fish contain mercury.[58] Limit the mercury in your body by avoiding higher-mercury fish, such as swordfish, king mackerel, and Chilean sea bass. The body eliminates the metal through the urine, so drink lots of water.

Lead

Dust, old paint, corroding pipes, and certain hobbies can lead to the inhalation or ingestion of lead. It replaces the calcium in your body, which affects your mind because neurons in the brain use calcium to communicate. Lead stays in the body for decades and causes nerve damage and high blood pressure. Iron deficiency correlates with high lead levels, so eating foods rich in iron, calcium, and vitamin B can help combat the effects of lead exposure.

DECLINE OF THE ROMAN EMPIRE

The neurotoxins in lead may have contributed to the dissolution of the Roman Empire. Ancient Romans drank wine from lead cups, and they fashioned the metal into pretty much everything they used: pipes, pots, utensils, even a common sweetener containing lead acetate. Researchers believe that the water they drank contained levels of lead 60 times higher than what the EPA allows.

Arsenic

A naturally occurring element, arsenic exists in the soil and rocks across most of America and many other countries. From there, it percolates into groundwater, which has a domino effect on fish, crops, and livestock. Even trace quantities in the body can interfere with your tumor-suppressing hormones, so arsenic exposure correlates with a variety of cancers. It harms lung cells and creates inflammation in the heart. The World Health Organization (WHO) estimates that at least 140 million people in 50 different countries are drinking water with damaging levels of arsenic.[59] In addition to testing your water, consuming dark, leafy greens, high-fiber foods, and lots of clean water can help flush arsenic from your system.

Heavy Metal Testing

If you experience symptoms of heavy metal poisoning, your doctor may order a heavy metal blood test, but you also can get a urine test to do at home without a doctor's order. A heavy metal blood test looks for the concentration of potentially hazardous metals in the bloodstream. Lead, mercury, arsenic, and cadmium are the most commonly examined metals. Copper, zinc, aluminum, and thallium are some of the less commonly tested metals.

TAKE ACTION

- The next time you (expect to) experience jet lag, get plenty of rest, take melatonin at the appropriate time, try a sleeping app or brain wave device, and drink lots of water.

- Avoid eating late at night, which can cause indigestion.

- For a better night's sleep and healthier weight, keep your sleeping space dark and no electronics in bed. If you can't avoid electronics, use blue light or nighttime filters on screens after sunset. If you can't avoid blue light at night, wear an eye mask to sleep.

- If you take prescription medication, follow timing instructions to the letter.

- Avoid excess caffeine, napping, and alcohol for a better night's rest.

- Set an alarm to remind you to go to sleep.

- Make a habit of not hitting snooze on your wake-up alarm.

- Investigate or create playlists of soundscapes designed to increase focus or relaxation.

- Delay or skip breakfast for a couple days and note your eating habits for the rest of those days.

- If you think you have a food sensitivity or allergy but haven't received a formal diagnosis, ask your physician for a referral to an allergist.

- To understand how the food you eat, the time you eat it, and how much you exercise affect your sugar levels, monitor your glucose levels closely for 30 days.

7.

THE POWER OF HABITS

"To keep the body in good health is a duty, otherwise we
shall not be able to keep our mind strong and clear."

—BUDDHA

WHEN I WAS A KID, MY PARENTS HAD A CHECKBOOK. AT THE END OF EVERY
month, they balanced it, tracking deposits and withdrawals to
make sure their totals matched the bank's records. When I was 12
years old, shopping with my parents, I spied a *Batman* toy. I had
seen *Batman* on television and desperately wanted that toy. I begged
my mom to buy it, but she said she didn't think we could afford it.
She told me to ask my father if he had enough cash to pay for it.

My father adored *Batman* as much I did, but he said he didn't
have the money then. He told me that maybe I'd get it for Christmas. I sulked the entire way home. Back at our house, my mother
asked me to put something into a closet. Inside, I noticed several
checkbooks that my father had stashed away. I ran up to him with
one of them in hand and said, "Look, Daddy, you have all of these
checks, and you told me you didn't have any money!"

He patiently explained that checks are a promise, not a guarantee. He had to have the money in the bank in order to write a
check. If all the money wasn't there, the check would bounce, and

the bank would charge him a fee, further depleting his account. "You can't spend what you don't have," he said time and again.

Our bodies are bank accounts. We have to balance them, and we also have to make sure we have what we need before we spend it fighting infections or diseases. That balancing act is called homeostasis. As you age, understanding what maintains your balance becomes increasingly important to improve your chances of long-term survival. Good balance allows you to live a longer life and continue doing what you enjoy for years to come.

HOMEOSTASIS

The internal systems of all living things, from plants to puppies to people, must maintain a stable state to process nutrients and distribute the results accordingly, much like making a bank deposit and then using it to pay bills. Each organism uses different mechanisms, but the goal remains the same: maintain homeostasis and survive.

If your blood pressure skyrockets or your body temperature plummets, your systems, organs, and cells may struggle to function. If that imbalance goes uncorrected, health decay ensues, and organs malfunction or fail. If your lungs lack oxygen for as few as 4 minutes, you can die. Even if you don't die, oxygen deprivation can kill brain cells in a matter of minutes. If a blockage stops blood from reaching your heart, a heart attack results. Those are major disruptions, but even small ones can cause big health problems.

In the 19th century, Claude Bernard, the father of modern experimental physiology, discovered that pancreatic secretions contained digestive enzymes. In doing so, he posited that (translated from the French) "the stability of the internal environment is the requirement for a free, independent life." Walter Cannon, a physiologist and one of the world's greatest scientists, built on Bernard's work, coining the word "homeostasis" in the early 1920s

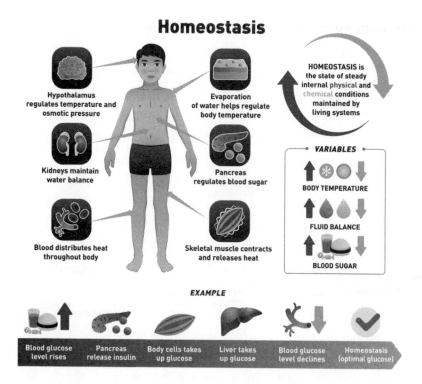

Homeostasis

Hypothalamus regulates temperature and osmotic pressure

Evaporation of water helps regulate body temperature

HOMEOSTASIS is the state of steady internal physical and chemical conditions maintained by living systems

Kidneys maintain water balance

Pancreas regulates blood sugar

VARIABLES

BODY TEMPERATURE

Blood distributes heat throughout body

Skeletal muscle contracts and releases heat

FLUID BALANCE

BLOOD SUGAR

EXAMPLE

| Blood glucose level rises | Pancreas release insulin | Body cells takes up glucose | Liver takes up glucose | Blood glucose level declines | Homeostasis (optimal glucose) |

from the ancient Greek words for "similar" and "state of stability." In *The Wisdom of the Body*, Cannon describes how the body teems with "pulses of energy, so minute that very delicate methods are required to measure them." Much of Cannon's research remains relevant today, especially his explanations about how bodily systems work.

For our purposes, medical homeostasis means balance in:

- the salts, minerals, proteins, and other molecules in your blood and urine;
- the concentrations of hydrogen, calcium, potassium, sodium, glucose, carbon dioxide, and oxygen available to your cells;
- internal temperature, pH, and other metrics.

Hydrogen, for example, helps you maintain a constant pH and

temperature. Your circadian rhythm lowers your body temperature at night. But if you're sick, your body produces a fever. As you can see, maintaining equilibrium requires a complex symphony of chemistry, physiology, and physics that takes place during every second of your life. In healthy people under normal conditions, these processes occur constantly. Imagine if you continuously had to tune your body's temperature like a finicky manual thermostat or measure your pH levels hundreds of times a day. Your body does that automatically every second of the day.

To achieve homeostasis, multiple systems—immune, digestive, and others—frequently work together. The microbiota in your digestive system maintain your gut health and help your immune system prevent conditions such as inflammatory bowel disease. (As we saw previously, microbiome imbalance can lead to chronic intestinal inflammation.)

Allostatic Overload

Your body's adaptive process that adjusts your homeostasis as needed is called allostasis. For example, when you're sleeping, your heart rate and blood pressure remain low. If you wake up and go for a jog, your heart rate and blood pressure rise, adjusting for the new stress load.

Allostatic overload happens as the cumulative effect of health-damaging behaviors and stress. If you don't get enough sleep for several weeks or you smoke three packs of cigarettes a day for 10 years, you're putting your system under incredible stress. Traumatic events, high-stress jobs, and even struggling with poverty cause wear and tear in any body system. Over time, the body's constant struggle to regain homeostasis results in allostatic overload, which can contribute to cardiovascular disease, depression, diabetes, hypertension, obesity, and other critical illnesses. Estimates peg stress as playing a role in 50 to 70 percent of all physical illnesses.[60]

The immune system contributes to homeostasis by giving the

body what it needs to fight infections or heal after trauma. If you sustain a cut, your mast cells release chemicals that bring more oxygen and immune cells to the injury. Macrophages eat the dead and broken cells and release a protein that causes new blood vessels and skin to form. In this case, the immune system helps your skin restore homeostasis. If the immune system fails, infections can worsen and spread, which commonly happens when unnoticed tooth infections migrate to the heart.

The human body can repair itself, but everyone's ability to cope with biological and physiological threats varies, especially given our different diets and lifestyles. But you can help your body to maintain homeostasis and a healthy immune system with better lifestyle habits.

External Factors

Doctors often call your personal habits "external factors," with the body being the internal factor. That's too simplistic, though. Your longevity relates directly to good physical and mental health. The problem is that we're getting sicker each year. In America, a large number of patients require medical attention for a variety of health conditions all occurring at the same time, a situation called "multimorbidity." Comorbidity means having more than one illness in a person at the same time—diabetes and congestive heart failure, for instance. Multimorbidity means more than two illnesses at once.

BAD HABITS

Many people constantly take omeprazole for acid reflux or use diphenhydramine (Benadryl) to fall asleep every night, counteracting bad habits—eating the wrong foods, drinking too much caffeine—with more bad habits. Two wrongs don't make a right.

A 25-year study of the National Health and Nutrition Examination Survey found that 59.6 percent of all adults have more than two multimorbidities, a number that has increased by 12 percent since 1988.[61] That number also stands poised to increase further as more people deal with the COVID virus and its respiratory and cardiac fallout.

Most of these conditions are preventable, and harmful daily habits exacerbate them. That means that, with time and effort, you can slow down and even reverse the aging process. Daily habits that prevent health decay, stave off disease, and optimize your body's systems can make a massive difference in how well you live. You can control those "external" factors and truly change your life.

LIFE EXPECTANCIES

Since 1995, obesity and diabetes have risen to epidemic levels in America. Unhealthy life habits, such as consuming sugar and carbohydrates in excess, can lead to immune system malfunctions over time, which shortens your life. A study by the UK Office for National Statistics found that a girl born in 2019 is expected to live 3 *fewer* years than a girl born in 2014. In that study, boys born in 2019 are expected to live about 1 fewer year than their 2014 counterparts.[62] The AHA warns that one in three children and teens in the United States are overweight, obese, or severely obese, putting them at greater risk for diabetes, stroke, cancer, asthma, and other diseases.[63] Today's children may live shorter, less healthy lives than their parents.

Biotech companies are delving into understanding the biology of aging to create new products and medications. But doctors and clinical researchers have known for decades that bad habits correlate with illness. Choices become habits, and habits become patterns. You choose every day whether to create good patterns or bad. Let's look at several habits that you can improve easily.

NUTRITION

With the rise of agribusiness and the explosion of fast, processed foods, it's easy to forget that food is supposed to fuel your body, maintain your health, and prevent disease, not satisfy cravings. Food gives your cells information and communicates with your organs. The quality of what you eat becomes even more important when you have special needs. For people who are recovering from an infection, pregnant, or lactating, consuming the right nutrients vitally restores homeostasis and boosts the immune system.

As you learn more about the science of food and nutrition, you'll have to examine your own food beliefs carefully and decide what changes you want to make. As always, discuss any dietary changes with your healthcare provider, particularly if you have other health concerns. We'll delve more deeply into good food habits later, but let's highlight a few here.

Eat foods high in anthocyanins, the chemical compounds that make fruits and veggies—such as blackberries, blueberries, carrots, cauliflower, and corn—purple. Anthocyanins provide protection from DNA damage, boost cytokine production, and have anti-inflammatory properties. Consume lots of bioflavonoids, which offer similar benefits as anthocyanins and occur in black tea, citrus, cocoa, and parsley. Take vitamin D and A supplements to boost your immune system. Vitamin A, when used correctly, can support the body's ability to fight respiratory infections. Pursue diversity, especially when it comes to grains (oats and barley) and mushrooms. If you don't already, incorporate nutritional yeast, spirulina, and seaweed into your diet. Processed, packaged foods never deliver the same nutritional value, no matter what claims manufacturers slap on the labels.

On its website, a popular brand of egg substitute touts itself as "plant-based eggs." But plants don't lay eggs. A closer look reveals more than 20 ingredients, including tetrasodium pyrophosphate, an inorganic compound that, when ingested orally, has a toxicity level approximately twice that of table salt. This product also contains transglutaminase, which occurs naturally in the body as a microbial enzyme. The food industry uses it to bind proteins together and to extend a product's shelf life. In that capacity, transglutaminase has links to celiac disease. If nature didn't make it, don't take it.

THE 10-INGREDIENT RULE

Food companies often use a trick in advertising, claiming that their products are "made from plants" or "whole" to make you think the product is organic, natural, or healthy. Look at the label, though. If you can't pronounce an ingredient, it probably came from a lab, not a farm. If a product has more than 10 ingredients, make sure that at least 7 are natural and organic.

Food Elements

It's important to understand the science of nutrition. If you have any special dietary needs, discuss them with your healthcare provider before making any dietary changes. Food nourishes the human body, but it's much more than that. It satisfies your needs for energy, structure, regulation, and protection. You should understand the main food elements to comprehend their relationship with your body.

Carbohydrates

Whether simple or complex, this macronutrient provides energy to your cells. Carbs not used right away become glycogen or convert to fat stored for future energy needs.

Fats

These super-concentrated energy sources, also a macronutrient, carry fat-soluble vitamins and serve as sources of essential fatty acids. If consumed in excess, they also convert to body fat for future use.

Proteins

Especially important to your immune system, this third macronutrient plays a key role in the production of enzymes, hormones, and antibodies. Proteins rich in casein from dairy or albumin from eggs help form new tissues as well as maintain and repair those already formed. When consumed to excess, protein converts to carbohydrates and fats for future needs.

Vitamins and Minerals

These micronutrients, such as calcium, iodine, iron, phosphorus, potassium, and sodium (minerals), drive the proper function of your immune cells every day. They also regulate bodily processes, from blood clotting to nerve stimuli. Fat-soluble vitamins include A, D, E, and K; water-soluble vitamins include B and C. Each contributes to the immune system in a variety of ways, including protecting healthy cells, promoting the growth and activity of immune cells, and stimulating the production of antibodies.

According to epidemiological studies, malnourished people have a greater risk of contracting bacterial, viral, and other infections because even just a single nutrient deficiency can harm immune response—but particularly deficiencies in zinc, selenium, iron, folic acid, copper, and B vitamins.

Supplements

For decades, the medical community has been divided over whether the body requires supplements. Some doctors advocate for proactive supplementation, but others strongly oppose it. Our bodies have built-in detoxification systems, including the kidneys and liver, which is good because we're consuming more synthetic chemicals than ever before. Our ancestors faced air pollution from fires, but not global contamination, and bacteria, but not antibiotic-resistant strains. We also have to contend with heavy metals, pesticides, processed foods, and more that their bodies never encountered. At the same time, poor eating habits are preventing us from getting enough salts and minerals. Supplementing your diet with vitamins, minerals, and adaptogens can help your body excrete the chemicals and viruses, such as HPV, that have been lingering inside your system for months, sometimes years.

Specific supplements can help certain conditions. Adults with osteoporosis, for example, may require more vitamin D and calcium that what they obtain from their diets. According to some studies, a combination of vitamin C, vitamin E, carotenoids, zinc, and copper can slow the course of age-related macular degeneration, a leading cause of visual loss in the elderly. People with Crohn's disease or celiac disease, which make it difficult to absorb certain nutrients, may benefit from supplements. A vitamin B_{12} deficiency, common for many people, almost always necessitates supplementation. Supplements that replenish depleted metabolites and help create new mitochondria can boost your metabolism. As you age, mitochondrial decline causes your metabolism, the process by which your body turns food into energy, to become less efficient. For your immune system, the choices become less clear. Companies are developing comprehensive immunological support in a daily supplement. As part of my professional research, I have analyzed 50 different "immune booster" supplements, but no products currently available in America have met my expectations.

Some supplements function best when taken with others. For example, if you want to slow the aging process, taking a daily complement that provides mitochondrial support as well as cellular renewal can be a good idea. For brain health and clarity, a daily complex with nootropics can supercharge your gray matter and slow the pace of cognitive decline.

People with allergies, known or undiscovered, should exercise caution about what they take. Supplements often include dairy products or derivatives as well as PUFAs and vegetable oils that are bad for you.

Adaptogens

Sourced from herbs or mushrooms, adaptogens enable your body to adapt to physical, chemical, or biological stress. According to theory, they boost "nonspecific" resistance to negative influences on the body, activating the body's stress-response mechanism and helping restore homeostasis. Used for millennia in Ayurvedic medicine, with scientific studies confirming their benefits, common adaptogens include ashwagandha, bilberry, ginseng, lion's mane, and reishi mushrooms. They do have a number of proven health benefits, including the ability to improve cellular function, brain activity, and the immune system. They come as tinctures, teas, powders, and pills that you can take separately or together.

Buyer Beware

According to a 2017 survey of 3,500 people aged 60 or older published in the *Journal of Nutrition*, 70 percent of those polled took a daily supplement (multivitamin or an individual micronutrient), 54 percent took one or two supplements, and 29 percent took four or more.[64] In America alone, OTC supplements generate annual revenue of around $30 billion. So are they worth it or a waste of money?

Not all supplements are created equal, and there's no one-size-fits-all answer for individual needs. Most manufacturers combine good ingredients with harmful additives or vegetable oils, so it's important to know what you're buying. Oils derived from plants such as corn, oil palms, safflowers, soybeans, and sunflowers often go into car and other industrial lubricants. Supplement manufacturers use them to extend shelf life.[65] Your heart, arteries, and other systems don't need them, and consuming them can disrupt the mechanisms that keep you healthy.

If you eat a well-balanced diet, you shouldn't need supplements. But who nowadays can adhere, around the clock, to a truly healthy diet that excludes alcohol and chemicals? You can't avoid hidden toxins like skipping wine with dinner. Supplements aren't a substitute for a healthy, well-balanced diet, nor are they a cure-all, but they can help you regain balance, especially when combined with better lifestyle habits such as drinking good-quality water, drinking less or no alcohol, eating less ultraprocessed food, and reducing the sugar content in your diet.

SUGAR

According to research, the quickest way to develop type 2 diabetes is to consume six packages of candy per day while sipping on a fizzy sweet beverage. That may sound extreme, but plenty of people do exactly that—sometimes or even often. Just one sugary soda can impact your immune system for hours after you drink it. Sugar damages your innate immune system, and too much sugar in your system allows bacteria and viruses to thrive. That's why people with diabetes have a greater risk for infections and gangrene.

A study in the *American Journal of Clinical Nutrition* found that it took only 75 grams of sugar to weaken the immune system. One sugary soda and one candy bar, together, have that sugar content. After you consume them, it takes your system several hours to recover—assuming you don't ingest more sugar. Even if you do everything right—sleeping 8 hours a night, exercising regularly, eating right—you still can harm your immune system with a couple of sodas or candy bars.

Many forms of sugar are natural, meaning grown and not manufactured, so "all-natural" products can contain tons of sugar. Also, anything in an ingredient list that ends in *-ose* is a kind of sugar. Food companies sometimes sneak more in there with multiple -oses, including dextrose, fructose, galactose, glucose, and maltose.

Sugar Synonyms

Common substitutes and synonyms for sugar include agave nectar, agave syrup, barley malt, beet sugar, blackstrap molasses, brown rice syrup, brown sugar, buttercream, cane juice, cane sugar, caramel, carob syrup, castor sugar, coconut sugar, confectioners' sugar, corn syrup, corn syrup solids, crystalline fructose, date sugar, Demerara sugar, dextrin, dextrose, diastatic malt, ethyl maltol, Florida Crystals, fructose, fruit juice, fruit juice concentrate, galactose, glucose, glucose syrup solids, golden sugar, golden syrup, grape sugar, high-fructose corn syrup, honey, icing sugar, invert sugar, lactose, malt syrup, maltodextrin, maltose, maple syrup, molasses, muscovado sugar, panela sugar, raw sugar, refiner's syrup, rice syrup, sorghum syrup, Sucanat, sucrose, treacle, turbinado sugar, and yellow sugar.

ALCOHOL

According to neuroscience, no amount of alcohol is safe for brain function. Scientists, researchers, and clinicians have studied the link between alcohol consumption and health decay for a long time. Because of alcohol's effects on innate and adaptive immunity, chronic drinkers predispose themselves to a wide range of health problems.

As it passes through the body, alcohol first contacts the gastrointestinal system, which absorbs it into your bloodstream. Alcohol alters the numbers and variety of microbes in the gut biome. These disruptions can impede your ability to fight infection, cause organ damage, and slow tissue recovery. Most everyone knows that excessive alcohol consumption can harm the liver, which processes toxins. But alcohol also damages the fine hairs inside the lungs that keep pathogens out of the airway. In addition to that, it impairs the immune cells in key organs, including the lungs, making you more vulnerable to respiratory illnesses. That double whammy creates a recipe for pulmonary disaster.

But that's not all. A study published in the March 2022 issue of *Nature* found that one drink a day can shrink the overall volume of your brain. On average, people over age 50 who drank a pint of beer daily had brains that appeared 2 years older than those who drank half a beer. Each additional drink per day contributed to the premature aging of their brains.[66]

Pregnant women who drink dramatically increase their newborn's risk of infection and disease, such as fetal alcohol syndrome. Alcohol use by the mother impacts a baby's immune system, and new evidence suggests that those negative effects last into adulthood.[67]

Drinking the least amount of alcohol possible gives you the best strategy for strong immunity and disease prevention.

HANGOVER HELPERS

If you overindulge, don't take acetaminophen (Tylenol) for any aches or pains, as it can damage your liver further. Aspirin, ibuprofen, or naproxen is OK. Also take vitamin B complex, which helps your body metabolize the alcohol and its by-products still in your system, and milk thistle, which helps your liver heal after it processes all those toxins.

EXCESS WEIGHT

If you're consuming the wrong foods, including sugar and alcohol, you probably weigh more than you should. Some studies have found that a large waistline increased the risk for women dying of cardiovascular disease, even when they were considered normal weights by body mass index (BMI) measurements.[68]

Obesity correlates with low-grade, chronic inflammation, which stresses your immune system. Fat tissue produces adipocytokines, which can promote inflammation. Research on the topic continues, but obesity also appears to be a risk factor for the flu virus, possibly due to the impaired function of T cells.[69] According to the latest research, too much or too little body fat can degrade your immune system. Excess weight and the accompanying inflammation can put you at risk of developing type 2 diabetes, hypertension, and heart disease.

If your doctor tells you that you need to lose weight for better health, follow that directive.

STRESS

When stressed, your body produces cortisol, which lowers your ability to fight infections, making you more vulnerable to whatever pathogens come your way. In as little as 30 minutes, anxious thoughts can weaken your immune response because that stress has disrupted your body's homeostasis.

When you encounter a perceived threat—a horror movie, a large animal coming toward you, an intruder in your house—your hypothalamus activates an alarm throughout your body. Your adrenal glands, which sit atop each of your kidneys, secrete a flurry of hormones, including adrenaline and cortisol, to help you handle whatever is happening. Adrenaline spikes your heart rate, blood pressure, and energy levels. Cortisol, the primary stress hormone, raises glucose levels in the bloodstream, improves the brain's ability to process glucose, and increases your body's capacity to repair its tissues. Cortisol also suppresses functions unnecessary or harmful in situations of fight, flight, or freeze. It subdues the digestive system, reproductive system, and even the growth process, allowing your body to focus on dealing with the stressor. This alarm system also communicates with the parts of the brain that control happiness, motivation, and fear.

Under chronic stress, your body maintains persistently high levels of cortisol, which correlate with increased appetite and weight gain. Too much stress can lead to binge eating unhealthy snacks or excessive alcohol consumption, both of which can cause nutritional deficiencies and a weakened immune system. That's why maintaining cortisol balance is so essential to homeostasis. Cortisol is your body's emergency department, there for momentary crises but not a substitute for daily good habits. If you can't shake your anxiety or if it interferes with daily life, talk to your doctor, a therapist, or both.

The COVID pandemic put added stress on virtually everyone. We had to live in isolation, but we humans are social creatures, so that seclusion may have taken a toll on our mental health as much as our physical well-being. You may have experienced fear, grief, financial hardship, or all of those during the pandemic, which only compounds stress. As a result, many people probably aged more quickly during the pandemic than they otherwise would have, a strange-sounding reality supported by scientific evidence. Stress causes inflammation in the body, which eventually shortens your telomeres, which accelerates aging.

The Lingering Effects of Isolation

When the SARS coronavirus ripped across the world, I was living in San Francisco, conducting early-phase clinical trials on breakthrough immunotherapies for cancer patients. We were fighting for survival while also dodging a deadly, changing virus. We who survived had our lives turned upside down and quickly learned how broken our medical systems had become. As an immunologist, I couldn't just watch from the sidelines as the world fell apart. From those early days of outbreaks, I involved myself in several projects aimed at helping the pandemic response.

After the pandemic restrictions began lifting, one of my

friends had to go back to the office. She went, came home, crawled into the shower, and sobbed for hours. What used to matter—her career and climbing the corporate ladder—didn't anymore. The stress of battles that she no longer wanted to fight hit her hard. Too often, we soldier on instead of dealing with what quite literally is making us sick, and as we all experienced firsthand, quarantine stress is very real. A study in *The Lancet* found that just 9 days of quarantine can raise stress levels in adults and children.[70]

Managing stress by reducing its triggers—toxic thoughts, places, people—can help unlock the secrets to better immune health. Everyone experiences stress differently, so you can decrease it in a variety of ways, including breathing exercises, meditation or prayer, and other methods that we'll review in Part Three.

EXERCISE

Regular physical activity can improve your sleep, metabolic balance, and memory. But exercising at the wrong time of the day can cause more harm than you might imagine. Remember those circadian rhythms? It turns out that your internal clock also influences exercise. Different cells, tissues, and organs have different sensitivities to exercise, depending on the time of day.

You may prefer an afternoon run or an evening workout class, but research has shown that morning is the best time for strenuous physical activity. That's when your cortisol levels are at their highest. Jawbone, a maker of wireless headsets and fitness trackers, conducted a study of 1 million people, analyzing their workout habits. The study found that people who exercise in the morning are more likely to work out three or more times a week, the recommended rate. Of the participants, 11 percent exercised at 6 a.m., the most popular hour, with 5 a.m. coming in second place. Late sleepers preferred a 9 a.m. start. People who hit the gym at 6 p.m. tended to have more inconsistent regimens.[71]

Different tissues respond to exercise at different times of the day, but those responses connect to create an orchestrated response that controls your body's overall energy levels. It improves your mood, boosts your energy, and helps you sleep better. Exercise acts as an appetite suppressant, which can help control your weight, and it combats many health conditions. Despite all that great science, only a quarter of Americans get regular exercise. That number hasn't changed in the last 20 years, despite continued public awareness campaigns about the multitude of benefits of physical activity.[72]

Moderate Movement

Recent studies have shown that, if you're not careful, high-intensity interval training (HIIT), a recent craze in the fitness world, can harm your immune system as well as your cartilage.[73] Low-intensity slow-state (LISS) exercise, on the other hand, can boost your immune system.

Jogging and other weight-bearing activities strengthen your muscles and bones. Strong bones help prevent osteoporosis and fractures later in life. Strength or resistance training—lifting weights, for example—can benefit your overall health because it helps you maintain muscle mass. Muscle is denser than fat, though, so it may cause your weight to rise slightly. As with anything, too much isn't good. Too much lifting can harm your knees, elbows, and back and accelerate wear and tear on your cartilage as well.

Regular moderate exercise improves your cardiovascular health, lowering your risk of type 2 diabetes and metabolic syndrome (hypertension, high blood sugar, excess body fat, abnormal cholesterol or triglyceride levels, and other symptoms). Exercise reduces the incidence of certain cancers, such as breast and colon cancer.

It improves your mood and sharpens your thinking and judgment. Best of all, it improves your ability to stay engaged, to reap the benefits of vitality, and to prolong your life. According to the CDC, people who exercise for about 7 hours a week have a 40 percent lower risk of dying prematurely than those who exercise for fewer than 30 minutes a week.[74]

Rest

Downtime between workouts allows the body to recover from and adapt to previous exertion. Exercise depletes your body's energy resources and hydration, so you need to time to replenish those stores. Maintaining an adequate supply of muscle glycogen, the body's carbohydrate store, is critical for keeping blood-sugar levels consistent. Several studies have found that the body needs at least 24 hours to restore spent muscle glycogen. Recovering your fluids takes less time, only 1 to 2 hours. But due to the ongoing production of urine, your body still requires more time to return to good hydration.

Muscles require several weeks of exertion and recovery cycles in order to grow, a cycle called physiological adaptation. Muscle, tendon, and ligament turnover happens at a rate of 0.4 to 1.2 percent every day. When resting, your body has a chance to repair and create tissue. Longer-term adaptations, such as

---

TIME YOUR GAINS

To improve protein synthesis, researchers discovered that, during a 12-hour period, consuming whey protein every 3 hours was more efficient than either every 1½ or 6 hours.[75]

---

increasing your number of blood vessels or growing the size of your heart, take months of training and rest. Whatever your goals, sticking with a regular routine of exercise and rest will increase your aerobic capacity, making your entire body more efficient and stronger.

Rest days also help prevent overtraining syndrome, which can lead to injuries, weariness, insomnia, depression, weight gain, and (ironically) a halt in muscle growth. Sleep deprivation in particular will denigrate your physical fitness and overall health. A comprehensive study found that sleep deprivation can tire you more easily during your next workout, along with other unfavorable consequences for cognitive function.[76]

Exercise and Weight Loss

It's virtually impossible to sweat your way out of overeating, but burning energy can help you keep weight off after you've lost it. Let's look at the math.

It takes a deficit of about 3,500 calories to lose one pound. For every mile of running or walking, most people burn only about 100 calories. A nice piece of chocolate cake has around 400 or 500 calories. If you eat that piece of cake, you'd have to walk or run 4 or 5 miles just to break even, creating no deficit and losing no weight. If you don't eat the cake and burn a deficit of 500 calories per day, you'll lose that pound in a week. According to research on how your metabolism and brain adapt to diet and exercise, even a small amount of weight loss would necessitate a *lot* of exercise. If you exercise vigorously for long periods of time, as professional athletes do, you'll lose weight because your body is burning thousands of calories per day. But ordinary people don't and can't exercise like that, and if you do, you'll feel more hungry than usual because your body will try to maintain its metabolic homeostasis.

SLEEP

When it's time for you to sleep, your circadian clock sets the process in motion. Your circadian rhythms control many organs, including the brain. These rhythms follow cues from daylight, which makes you feel alert, and darkness, which makes you feel sleepy. Bright artificial light or stimulants, such as caffeine or alcohol, can increase alertness even at night, disrupting your clock and pushing it forward.

Your brain releases a variety of neurotransmitters that send signals to promote sleep or wakefulness. GABA, a neurotransmitter, reduces nerve cell activity, which is crucial for sleep. Adenosine, another neurotransmitter, accumulates in the brain during the day and, when it reaches high concentrations, makes you feel sleepy at night. Caffeine keeps you awake by blocking adenosine receptors in the brain. In response to darkness, your brain produces melatonin, a hormone. Light exposure, natural or artificial, inhibits melatonin production and increases the release of cortisol, which wakens you. When exposed to too much artificial light late at night, such as the blue light from electronic screens, your body produces less melatonin, making it more difficult to fall asleep. Serotonin, the "feel-good" neurotransmitter, plays a role in both sleep and wakefulness. The brain releases it by day and uses it to make melatonin at night.

At various points in your sleep-wake cycle, your brain also releases a variety of hormones, including adrenaline, cortisol, histamine, and norepinephrine, which counter sleep. Produced in response to stress, these hormones cause your body to wake and become more alert. Under chronic stress, your body produces adrenocorticotropic hormone (ACTH), which produces cortisol. Insomniacs have higher levels of ACTH.

When sleeping, your body goes through two main stages of

sleep: rapid eye movement (REM) and non-rapid eye movement (non-REM). Throughout an average night, you cycle through these phases around four to six times, and it's not uncommon to wake up briefly between cycles. You dream in REM sleep, which is important, but you spend the majority of your sleeping hours in non-REM sleep.

Not getting enough sleep or sleeping poorly could have one or more of several causes:

- drinking caffeinated or alcoholic beverages late in the day or evening
- watching television or using screens late at night
- not following a regular sleep schedule
- sleeping environment too bright, too loud, or otherwise unsuitable
- circadian time shifting, such as jet lag, working overnight, or pulling an all-nighter
- disorders, such as sleep apnea, insomnia, or periodic limb movements
- other medical conditions, including chronic pain or heart, lung, or kidney disease

Lack of sleep spikes your cortisol levels, which makes your immune system struggle to maintain homeostasis. Cortisol also breaks down the collagen in your skin, which causes premature wrinkles. Studies show that sleep deprivation harms your memory, motor skills, and brain. You have a greater likelihood of making mistakes or getting into a car accident when tired. Continued deprivation raises your risk of cardiovascular disease, cancer, depression, diabetes, and stroke. The last two bullets above require medical assessment and intervention, but you have the power to change the first five.

IGNORANCE

You're reading this book, so you're ahead of the game on this topic, but that doesn't mean you can stop paying attention. There's a lot to understand and consider about the chemicals you encounter, the foods you consume, the consequences of those love handles or that stressful job, and how all of that affects your body. But it all matters, especially if you want to slow the aging process and live a long, healthy life. Whether you're trying to understand the effects of chemicals in your drinking water, decoding labels at the grocery store, or deciding whether to have a glass of wine or go for a jog, remain vigilant and reliably informed. Your health is literally at stake. Whenever your body is malnourished, intoxicated, or otherwise suffering, it breaks down in ways both large and small. Your daily habits impact every part of your body, so carefully consider the decisions you make today and tomorrow. They might just save your life.

TAKE ACTION

- If you regularly take omeprazole, Benadryl, or OTC sleep aids, wean yourself off them.

- Pay attention to how much of your food comes from packages.

- Eat foods high in anthocyanins and bioflavonoids. Incorporate nutritional yeast, spirulina, or seaweed into your regular diet. Supplement with vitamins D and A. Diversify what you consume.

- Try to avoid store-bought foods containing more than 10 ingredients.

- If a single food that you're about to eat has more than 10 ingredients, make sure that at least 7 are natural and organic.

- Look at the foods that you eat regularly or keep stocked at home. Check the nutritional labels for added sugars and the ingredient lists for words ending in -ose.

- Reduce your alcohol intake. If you do drink, don't take acetaminophen to relieve a hangover. Take aspirin, ibuprofen, or naproxen instead, along with vitamin B complex and milk thistle.

- If anxiety or other manifestations of stress interfere with your daily life, make an appointment to talk to your doctor or a therapist.

- If you exercise inconsistently, try shifting your workouts or other physical activity to the morning or at least earlier in the day.

- If you exercise regularly, don't neglect to incorporate meaningful rest into your routine.

- Avoid stimulants, such as alcohol and caffeine, and blue light from electronic screens for better sleep.

- Keep asking yourself: Are my daily habits preventing disease or enabling it?

8.

THE FUTURE OF MEDICINE

"The future belongs to those who prepare for it today."

—Malcolm X

IN ANCIENT EGYPT, DURING THE EARLY DAYS OF MEDICINE, PRIESTS ALSO served as doctors. They practiced the earliest recorded forms of medicine at Houses of Life, or temples, along the Nile River. For thousands of years, the mysteries of science, biology, and human diseases appeared mystical. In more recent history, people who lived in small towns rarely drove to city hospitals for routine medical appointments. Urgent care clinics didn't exist. Instead, virtually all small towns had their own doctors who lived in the community. They knew every single resident, from birth or to death, and those personal connections allowed small-town doctors to personalize patient care.

Since the time of priest-doctors, we have made monumental advancements in medicine. We have discovered thousands of cell types, millions of genome variants, countless disease-associated genes, and an almost unimaginable number of ways in which they all can combine in your body. With every new piece of knowledge, we come closer to cracking the code for longer life.

But our current healthcare systems, as the medical community is acknowledging, largely fix problems when things go awry rather than proactively keeping people healthy. Over the last century, as bureaucracy and profit margins have overpowered the deeper principles of medicine, the human touch has faded. An ironic downside of new technology is that hyperpersonalized medical care often neglects the human component. That's why combining modern medicine with old-fashioned relationships is so important in doctor-patient associations. Switzerland in particular is making that movement, called personomics, a reality, and it has been gaining traction elsewhere around the world. Personomics uses the cutting-edge benefits of technology in concert with a greater understanding of the personal factors that shape a patient's health.

SOUNDING THE ALARM

A small-town doctor, Art van Zee had worked in the Pennington Gap, Virginia, community health clinic since the 1970s. In the late 1990s, he noticed an unusual number of opioid overdose deaths among teenagers in the town of 1,900 people. Dr. van Zee alerted Purdue Pharma to the problem and eventually petitioned for FDA involvement. Dr. van Zee's long-term relationships in the community gave him a frontline view of the coming opioid crisis.

PERSONOMICS

Precision medicine has many fields: epigenomics, or the study of what causes gene activation and deactivation; genomics, or the study of genomes; metabolomics, or the study of cellular metabolisms; and personomics and pharmacogenomics, which we'll explore in this chapter. The field of personomics looks at an individual's unique life circumstances and how those might influence disease susceptibility, genetic reaction to social decisions, and potential responses to different types of treatment. Depending on who practices it, personomics can incorporate behavioral, cultural, economic, mental, psychological, social, and even spiritual factors of any person into the overall healthcare equation.

What does that mean for you? By analyzing all of those circumstances and how they relate to your health, doctors can make more accurate predictions and help you navigate your way (back) to better health by analyzing more data points. Mapping different biomarkers against your work-life balance, for example, can help doctors determine what lifestyle changes you need to make as well as predict how well you will react to treatments.

NOT JUST NUMBERS

Your health consists of more than just lab results. It comes from what you consume, where you work, your community involvement, how much love you have in your life, and more. Social components greatly influence how well and how long you live. To get healthy, sometimes you need to revisit past choices, such as leaving a job you no longer enjoy or a relationship that has soured. Good health and long life require self-awareness, and only you can steer your own ship.

The influencer-driven attention economy encourages people to buy products, health-related or not, based on reviews or recommendations from like-minded individuals, who aren't necessarily experts. The weight loss plans, supplements, exercise routines, and adaptogens that your friend adores might do nothing for you, or worse, cause you harm. That's why personomic medicine is so effective. It aggregates all aspects of your life to create a 360-degree picture of your health. Then the data points to tailored solutions for everything from healthy aging routines to cancer treatments. You as a person are just as important to your own health as your DNA or lab test results.

This comprehensive approach is more than just a fad, though. It gives patients more autonomy while engaging and accounting for their social groups. The glut of information about even basic health decisions can feel confusing and overwhelming. Your doctor should help you navigate your choices, discuss potential treatment options, and answer your questions. When your doctor understands your cultural, community, and personal history, your chances of getting better care improve greatly.

If you ever have felt like just a number in the system, personomics aims to change that. Merging precision medicine with healthy living integrates different medical disciplines to have the greatest impact. Imagine, for example, combining data about your cardiorespiratory fitness and nutritional phenotype to improve heart health and manage your weight better. Personomics can rehumanize personalized medicine, and one of the best forms of personalized medicine pertains to the immune system.

IMMUNOTHERAPY

What if I told you that we can hack your immune system to combat diseases, including cancer? That's what immunotherapy does. I know because I've led and worked with Nobel Prize laureates on complex clinical trials for cancer patients using novel immunotherapy drug combinations. Immunotherapy is helping millions of people worldwide live longer, healthier lives. Some drugs can alleviate the painful symptoms of autoimmune diseases, such as psoriasis or rheumatoid arthritis. Others unleash the hidden powers of your immune system to shrink tumors in just days. It's not a one-size-fits-all solution, and scientists still struggle to understand why some patients' bodies resist treatment, but the future of the field looks bright.

It all started in the 1890s in New York City, when William Coley used a bacterium that causes a nasty skin infection to treat a patient with inoperable cancer. The patient, a man named Zola, had several advanced tumors, including one in his throat that prevented him from eating. Soon after Coley's treatment, the tumors shrank, and Zola went back to normal life. Today, medical ethicists would condemn such an experiment as totally unscrupulous, but Coley's trial proved successful and became one of the first known examples of immunotherapy. He later injected more than 1,000 cancer patients with bacteria or bacterial subproducts eventually called Coley's Toxins.

Back then, scientists considered the immune system a passive lump of functions that had little to do with treating disease. Coley came under heavy criticism because of his theories, but his principles were correct. Your immune system's capabilities go far beyond preventing infection. It has many untapped powers. Immunotherapy directs your body's natural defenses to fight diseases that have outwitted it. For example, if your body is rushing to fight a new bacterium, that army of immune cells can galvanize to fight a tumor.

At the time of Coley's Toxins, chemotherapy and radiation had just been developed, and doctors soon forgot about Coley's theories and work. But Coley still serves as a role model for the perfect doctor. Building on existing theories, he thought beyond the borders of existing common sense, treated patients, and analyzed only what he observed. His unconventional ideas helped deliver us to many of the discoveries we have today—thanks in no small part to other visionary scientists, who looked deeper into how the immune system can affect other areas of your health.

Nearly a century after Coley's work, the modern field of immunotherapy came into being. Many doctors, including myself, often go into specific areas of medicine because of loss in their own families. James Allison, the father of contemporary immunotherapy, watched his mother die of lymphoma and his brother of prostate cancer. Those struggles inspired Allison to pursue his life's work. In 1981, he suggested that the immune system had cancer-fighting abilities. In those days, the scientific community doubted even the possibility of treating and curing diseases by hacking the immune system. After many years of research, however, and with the help of many postdocs, interns, research nurses, and patients, he invented an immune checkpoint blockade. His research had revealed that one molecule in the body acted as the gas pedal for immune response, while another functioned as the brakes. Allison figured out how to override the brakes, giving the immune system a fighting chance at destroying the cancer.

From Allison's work, Bristol Myers Squibb developed ipilimumab under the brand name Yervoy. The first immune checkpoint blockade drug on the market, Yervoy extended the survival rate of patients with metastatic melanoma by several months to years, with 20 percent of patients living another decade or more. At the time, more than 50,000 people were dying of melanoma each year, according to the WHO. Other immune checkpoint blockade drugs have followed, and oncologists use them to fight bladder, kidney, lung, neck, skin, and other cancers.

Tasuku Honjo, a medical doctor and immunotherapy researcher, also made key contributions to the field. In the 1990s, still before the rise of conventional immunotherapy, Dr. Honjo's work identified a protein that plays a critical role in autoimmune diseases. In tests, inhibiting that protein enabled T cells to target and kill cancer cells. His discoveries aligned with Allison's research, and in 2018 Allison and Honjo jointly received the Nobel Prize in Medicine "for their discovery of cancer therapy by inhibition of negative immune regulation." Their work has revolutionized cancer treatment, saved countless lives, and changed our fundamental understanding of the immune system.

Around that same time, Allison teamed up with another researcher, Jeffrey Bluestone, to study T cells and their role in autoimmunity. In some autoimmune diseases, the immune system oversteps its mark. Bluestone and Allison identified a checkpoint that downregulates immune responses. The work of Bluestone and Allison helped uncover a secret interaction that cancer cells use to evade the immune system. That secret, when unveiled, brought immunotherapy as we know it into existence. Estimates put the market value of the field at more than $100 billion today.

Just like in your immune system, the field has two major branches: activation therapies, which enhance or stimulate your natural defenses, and suppressive therapies, which desensitize or subdue them.

Activation Immunotherapies

These therapies can fall into two categories: nonspecific, meaning they generate a general immune response, and specific, which generate responses targeting particular antigens. Different forms of activation immunotherapies include adoptive cell transfer, checkpoint inhibitors (which Allison used), targeted antibodies, tumor-infecting viruses, and vaccines.

Adoptive cell transfer uses a patient's own T cells, modifies and expands them in the lab, and then reinfuses them into the patient's body. Clinical studies have shown remarkable tumor regression in patients with metastatic melanomas who undergo this treatment.

Targeted antibodies, also called monoclonal antibodies, help protect against bacteria and viruses and can disrupt cancer cells, alerting the immune system to eliminate them. It took decades for the first monoclonal antibody drug for use in humans to come to market. In recent years, additional drugs have received approval for treating multiple diseases, and clinical researchers are developing hundreds more.

Viral infection immunotherapy has sent leukemia in some patients into remission. In the 1960s, researchers used viruses such as dengue, Epstein-Barr, and hepatitis to treat some types of cancer, but the poorly documented results varied. Those viruses didn't always work, but adenoviruses—which can cause bronchitis, conjunctivitis, croup, and pneumonia—showed more promising results. In one study at the time, clinicians treated 30 women who had advanced ovarian cancer with an adenovirus. Within 2 weeks, two-thirds of them showed tumor reduction.[77] Today, biotech companies are using viruses to prevent and treat diseases associated with cancer and even other viruses.

Vaccines have helped shaped our adaptive immunity since 1796, when Edward Jenner developed the first one, for smallpox, in Britain. Since then, vaccines have saved hundreds of millions of lives worldwide. As we learned in 2020, developing and testing mRNA vaccines for SARS-CoV-2 required monumental efforts by scientists, drug makers, and government agencies. Thankfully they succeeded. By eliminating several steps of the existing process, genomic vaccines promise even faster manufacturing times, and several clinical trials are testing them now. Biotech companies also are working to develop a single vaccine capable of addressing several diseases at once by coding sequences of multiple proteins and modifying them to address mutations and variants.

Suppressive Immunotherapies

Suppressing the immune system might sound like a bad idea at first, but it has a lot of helpful, practical benefits. The two biggest: transplants and life-threatening allergies. Your immune cells constantly patrol your body, looking for foreign substances to attack and neutralize. People with tissue or organ transplants need immunosuppressive drugs to train their immune systems not to fight and damage those new tissues. Without these medications, their bodies can reject life-saving transplants. In addition to treating serious allergies, calming your body from overreacting to a harmless substance, suppressive immunotherapy also can treat grave autoimmune conditions, such as Crohn's disease, lupus, multiple sclerosis, rheumatoid arthritis, and ulcerative colitis.

Years ago, doctors used to treat psoriasis with awful coal–tar shampoo, but good things can happen when drug makers bet on bold research. Your immune system naturally produces a protein called tumor necrosis factor (TNF). Some people generate too much of it, though, which causes inflammation. In clinical trials, researchers observed the drug adalimumab's effectiveness in combating psoriasis and other autoimmune conditions by stopping TNF from attacking healthy cells, thereby reducing inflammation. Sold under the brand name HUMIRA—for "human monoclonal antibody in rheumatoid arthritis"—adalimumab generated almost $20 billion in revenue in 2020 alone.

Conquering Cancer

I have seen the power of immunotherapy firsthand with a friend, whom we'll call David. He and his wife, Cheryl (also not her real name), shared an uncommon magic. They had a connection that spiritualists call being soulmates and romantics call love. Born and raised in a small town in Texas, they met in high school and married on graduation day. David worked in sales for almost two decades, and his number one mission in life was to make Cheryl happy.

One Monday morning, as David was driving their daughters to school, he felt a sharp pain in his lower back. He blamed the old car he was driving, but the pain worsened during the next several weeks. Cheryl worried that he was taking too much ibuprofen (an NSAID) to deal with the pain and wanted him to see a doctor. He didn't think he could afford the downtime from work. He just wanted the pain to stop. Later that year, after Thanksgiving dinner, he felt a pain so intense that he couldn't get off the couch. Cheryl took him to the hospital.

After a week of blood tests, scans, and biopsies, doctors diagnosed him with prostate cancer. Prostate-specific antigens (PSAs) liquefy semen and allow sperm to swim freely. Doctors measure it to evaluate the presence of prostate cancer. High levels of PSA usually indicate more aggressive cases. David's levels were 10 times higher than average, and the disease had spread to his bones.

From that day, the lives of David, Cheryl, and their family changed forever. The news devastated them, but the oncologist offered them a glimmer of hope. He assured them that surgery, radiotherapy, and chemotherapy could help David manage the disease. If all went well, he could live a healthy life.

David worked for a large tech company and had an advantage that many Americans don't. He had good, reliable medical insurance. His plan covered most of the procedures, and doctors advised that he could keep working while undergoing treatment.

Two months after surgery, however, they received bad news. The tumor was spreading quickly, and they needed to act fast. After reviewing the pathology report, David's oncologist—a rising star from New York, recruited to Houston—transferred him to a world-class cancer center. David now had an award-winning team working on his case, but hormone treatment failed, chemotherapy didn't stop the cancer from growing, and the side effects blurred his mind. After 2 years, he had lost 15 pounds, looked unrecognizable to himself, felt exhausted, and was having daymares. When cancer spreads, it can press on nerve cells, causing extreme discomfort. At one point, the pain became so intense that David asked for sedation. Worst of all, he had run out of treatment options.

Breaking bad news to patients is one of the hardest tasks that physicians face. Oncologists deliver grim diagnoses every day, but no formal training or preparation makes that soul-crushing task any easier. The team advised David to put his affairs in order and spend his remaining time with loved ones. The family fell into despair. They had nothing to do now but wait for death.

Then, as he was on his way to a hospice, David received a phone call. "There's a human clinical trial opening next week that you might qualify for," the oncologist said. "There are no guarantees, but we think you should come in and give it a shot."

Before the call even ended, his wife spun the car around. She wasn't giving up. "This is it," she said. "We're going back."

Back at the cancer center, the oncologist told them about a Phase 1 trial studying the strategic combination of two immuno-therapy drugs. It would hack David's immune system and empower his immune cells to target the cancer cells.

Before immunotherapy, various cancer treatments cut out tumors via surgery, poisoned them with chemotherapy, or burned them with radiotherapy. Immunotherapy doesn't attack tumors directly, though. In David's case, it removed the emergency brakes from his own defenses, allowing his immune system to go to work.

Three weeks after the first infusion, David's tumor shrank, his pain levels reduced by 70 percent, and he smiled for the first time in months. A year later, doctors declared him cancer-free, and he has remained in remission ever since. Every month, Cheryl still sends a key lime pie to the man who told them about the clinical trial. She believes that her family experienced a miracle. For me, the miracle is that our understanding of the immune system cured David's cancer. Maybe we're both right.

Genetic Modifications

Sometimes a genetic mutation present at birth prevents a person's body from producing a protein required to stop bleeding. Hemophilia B, a relatively rare disease, occurs in 1 in approximately 25,000 male births, causing a blood disorder that results in easy bruising and bleeding that can lead to hemorrhaging and even death. People with this condition frequently struggle with lifelong anxiety and fear because any accident, no matter how minor, might prove fatal.

Recent genetic therapy functionally helped cure this condition— but not in the way that you might think. Scientists genetically modified a virus to carry the blueprints for making the absent protein to the liver. After just one infusion, according to research published in the *New England Journal of Medicine*, the livers of 9 of the 10 patients in the clinical trial started producing normal amounts of the protein, and the patients no longer required regular injections of the clotting factor that they lacked. Many questions remain, of course. How much will gene therapies like this cost? How will patients have access to them? Will efficacy rates hold over time? But the results offer cause for optimism.[78]

Preventing HIV

According to the WHO, cancer accounted for almost 10 million deaths in 2020, making it one of the leading causes of death worldwide. Scientific understanding of the connection between tumor growth and the immune system began in earnest in the 1980s, though, during the AIDS epidemic. HIV ravaged patients' adaptive immune systems—resulting in deaths from rare tumors, such as Kaposi sarcoma—but the patients' innate immune systems still protected them from more common cancers. Doctors wanted to understand how to hack the immune systems of people suffering with HIV-AIDS to make those systems more effective.

The global prevalence of HIV infections has risen steadily over the years, from 8.5 million in 1990 to 35 million in 2013, even as highly effective antiretroviral therapy resulted in a dramatic decline in mortality rates. As we saw in the chapter on living with viruses, the best cure is prevention. PrEP (pre-exposure prophylaxis) consists of a daily pill of antiviral medications that destroy the virus in the body before it can infect T cells and macrophages. Clinical trials have shown Truvada and Descovy, two of the name brands on the market, to be safe, with few side effects, and to reduce the risk of sexual acquisition by up to 99 percent if taken with high adherence. In an ideal world, all who want it would have access to PrEP, just like birth control.

Not for Everyone

In healthy people, the immune system behaves predictably, targeting abnormal cells while ignoring healthy ones. Not every patient responds to immunotherapy drugs, though, and immunologists and immunotherapists still struggle with why. In isolation and in a lab, cells and systems operate in pretty much the same way, but how they interact with other cells varies slightly—or significantly—in every person. Plus, some people suffer major side effects from a hyperactivated immune system, so maintaining the balance between a therapy's effectiveness and limiting those side effects poses a significant challenge.

With immunotherapy, only about 15 to 20 percent of patients achieve long-lasting results. Of the 5,000 people a day who receive a cancer diagnosis in America, only 40 percent will be eligible for checkpoint inhibitor immunotherapy. On average, however, fewer than 15 percent will see clinical benefits. Some studies show, paradoxically, that, at times, a person's response to immune treatment can *cause* tumors to grow and spread. The journal *Clinical Cancer Research* found that, in 8 of 155 patients on immunotherapy treatment, tumors worsened.[79]

In many cases, tumors also become resistant to immunotherapy drugs or combinations of drugs, which is why doctors often use immunotherapy in combination with chemotherapy, radiation, surgery, and other treatments. When metastasis occurs, the cellular environment changes drastically from where the primary cancer developed, essentially creating two cancer problems to solve simultaneously. Those variables and interactivities can cause T cells to malfunction in an unknown number of ways. Certain cancers, including prostate cancer, prove incredibly resistant to immunotherapy. So David really was one of the lucky ones.

It's enormously gratifying to see treatment give hope to patients fighting cancer, psoriasis, rheumatoid arthritis, or the SARS coronavirus. Finding reliable predictors of patient response remains the biggest challenge that researchers face. Doctors still lack good tools to determine which patients will benefit from clinical trials, and patient profiling for those treatments has made slow progress.

In America, only about 8 percent of cancer patients take advantage of those novel treatments. Volunteers enroll in thousands of clinical trials worldwide, helping scientists find answers to the mysteries of modern medicine, but we need more. Experimental therapies become cures only after volunteers sign up for testing, but right now, there are more drugs available to be tested than volunteers.

PHARMACOGENOMICS

This field of research studies how your genes affect how you respond to medications. For example, 10 percent of the Caucasian population has a genetic variation that makes it difficult for their bodies to metabolize thiopurines, drugs that treat acute lymphoblastic leukemia. Clinical trials already are making use of pharmacogenomics, which is on its way to becoming the norm. Pharmaceutical companies are developing new pharmacogenomics-based drugs and determining how to personalize older drugs. (Advances in pharmacogenetics can move more slowly because drugs take longer to secure approval than molecular and diagnostic tests.)

What X-rays were to the last century, genotyping will be to our century. Genetic testing will improve predictions about predispositions to diseases, onset timing, scope, and even severity, as well as which treatments or medications probably would be effective or harmful. But genotyping doesn't always correlate with how you respond to a medication, which is another reason that personomics is so important, taking into consideration your lifestyle, environment, community, and culture to design the ideal treatment for you.

ARTIFICIAL INTELLIGENCE IN MEDICINE

Do you want to live past age 100 in good health and pain-free? Personomics, immunotherapy, and artificial intelligence (AI) are helping that happen. Two decades ago, the collective field of medicine looked very different—consider all the advancements just in genetics, stem cells, technology, and data crunching—and in a decade or two from now, doctors will interact with patients in different ways.

Telemedicine existed in its infancy before the coronavirus pandemic, but touchless check-ins, temperature checks, and virtual health visits all have become commonplace in the last few years. Connected health, the tech model of healthcare delivery, brings together wireless, digital, electronic, and mobile health technologies. As a subset of personomics, its goal isn't to become less personalized but more so. The devices, services, and interventions directly serve your needs. Health-related data seamlessly cross platforms and specialties so that you receive more proactive and efficient care.

These are just a few of the innovative technologies that will continue to evolve, improve, and play larger roles in clinical laboratories around the world:

- secure cloud accounts to store test results, baseline DNA, and genetic profiles;
- large-scale genomic analysis initiatives to inform therapy decisions;
- CRISPR technology for diagnostic and therapeutic purposes;
- digital bed monitoring with provider alerts for patients with fall risks or susceptibility to bedsores.

Storing, sharing, and using all of this information properly will be key for allowing you to make more informed choices and for personalizing medical treatments effectively.

NEURAL INTERFACE TECHNOLOGIES

In the 1960s, the invention of the first cochlear implant to treat hearing loss gave birth to the world of neural interface technologies (NITs). The FDA approved deep-brain stimulation in 1997 for the treatment of tremors. More recent, experimental treatments aim to restore bodily function after paralysis or blindness.

Elon Musk launched Neuralink in 2016 with the goal of connecting human brains and AI through "ultra–high bandwidth brain-machine interfaces." Pager, a 9-year-old macaque monkey, played a game of *MindPong* with the help of Neuralink technology. An interface implanted in Pager's brain allowed him to control a digital joystick using only his mind. The Neuralink chip recorded

Pager's neural activity, fed the data into a decoder algorithm, and predicted Pager's intended hand movements in real time. The project intends to develop that technology to allow people with paralysis to use phones or computers solely through brain activity.

Bryan Johnson's Kernel is developing another NIT, an optical headset that records real-time brain activity by means of local changes in blood oxygenation. In 2018, researchers at the University of California, Berkeley invented neural "dust," millimeter-sized implantable wireless nerve monitors and stimulators. Scientists are testing these tiny sensors, dubbed "electroceuticals," as a treatment for neurological disorders such as epilepsy and paralysis. Recent years have seen a push toward noninvasive, wearable NITs, such as the wrist-worn CTRL-kit. Introduced in 2019, it uses differential electromyography, translating electrical impulses into actions, allowing you to control machines with your mind.

It may sound like the stuff of science fiction, but touch screens, geolocators, headsets, and other electronic devices already connect you to virtual worlds. NITs just take those connections and possibilities a step further. Imagine if a brain implant could prevent you from developing Alzheimer's or mitigate its terrible symptoms. That's not yet possible, but researchers and biotech companies are trying to achieve that end. Future medicine will take advantage of the already blurring lines between mind and machine with patches, chips, and devices that will interact with your central and peripheral nervous systems. Those NITs, not yet invented, will transform the existing boundaries of medicine and human reality. Concerns about access, ethics, privacy, and regulation rightly remain, however.

In the future, you'll know more about your own health than you thought possible today. Genetic testing and epigenetic monitoring already give you a potential snapshot of your future. With more and better information, you and your doctors can tailor decisions and treatments to prevent illness, remedy it, and extend your life. Future breakthroughs in genetics, immunology, AI, and data science will empower you with knowledge, resources, tools, and ideal care. The more you know about what's happening inside your body, the more you'll understand how your personal choices impact your health and how to adjust them for a healthier, longer life.

TAKE ACTION

- Ask your healthcare providers if they know about or practice personomic medicine.

- Revisit past life choices that might be affecting your health. Think objectively about your relationships, job, and even where you live. Does your significant other make you a stronger person? Does your boss or do your clients inspire you or drag you down? Do you need to move? If you could start again, what would you do differently? What would make your heart sing? Will changing any of those situations improve your health? Write it all down and create an action plan for positive change in your life.

- Look at your friends list, too. Would you trade lives with them? Do they support you? Do you just put up with them? Curate the list accordingly.

- Ask your physician about volunteering in clinical trials.

- Ask your healthcare providers what digital or AI initiatives they're embracing and how those can improve your health or well-being.

PART THREE

THE IMMUNITY SOLUTION PROTOCOL

PROGRAM OVERVIEW

YEARS AGO, AT A MEDICAL SYMPOSIUM IN SWITZERLAND, AN ONCOLOGIST AT a roundtable discussion in which I was participating said that taking care of the body is like caring for a vintage car. Whenever his car needed repairs, he took it to an expert mechanic at a trusted garage. If your car started making unusual noises and you had no idea what was causing them, you probably would bring it to a professional. You would explain what was happening and entrust a person or team to identify the problem and fix it. You should do the same with your body. If something isn't functioning properly, you need expert medical assistance. Successful leaders know that delegating projects and tasks to experts results in better outcomes. The same goes for taking care of your body. Don't try to Google your way out of a health problem. Even medical professionals go to other experts to address their own health issues.

Allow me to pivot to a related metaphor. The hardware of your body allows your life to happen by means of components, the organs of your cardiovascular, respiratory, immune, and other systems. The software of your genetic code runs it all, and you are the user, the thinker trying to navigate and interact with your environment. While you're doing that, consciously directing your body, your systems and software work in the background to keep everything running as smoothly as possible.

But many people today often ignore the error messages that their systems generate to warn that something's wrong. Maybe you don't know why your gut is making that strange noise, or maybe you can't remember the last time you felt good. We let our everyday lives—hectic work schedules, family obligations, a general rush to get from A to B—sidetrack or interfere with our health. Down the road, the resulting burden may be physical as well as financial because healthcare can be expensive.

This step-by-step action plan, which will help you optimize your immune system, improving your overall health, begins with establishing baseline knowledge about your body and gives you a working template for daily and weekly routines that will keep your health in tip-top condition. The program lasts just 7 weeks, a mere blip in your entire life, but it can have powerful consequences. It gives you tools to boost your energy levels, avoid disease, slow the aging process, and live longer. You'll implement the steps gradually, one at a time, instead of making drastic changes overnight, and each subsequent week builds on the foundation and successes of the one before.

The first week, you'll get to know yourself, gathering health data and looking at where you stand right now. The second week, you'll learn about tracking tools so, as you develop healthier routines, you can monitor your progress. In the third week, when you start the Immunity Solution Diet, you'll explore the right eating habits for better immunity. The fourth week gives you practical techniques for sleeping better so that, in week five, you can move your body more effectively. You'll balance that physical activity with strategies in week six to calm your mind. In the final week, you'll fill any remaining gaps in your health with supplements (vitamins, minerals, adaptogens), and after that a maintenance guide will help you retain the benefits of the program long into the future.

Now let's get to work.

Week 1.

KNOW YOURSELF

JUST AS WITH A CAR, COMPUTER, OR SMARTPHONE, YOU CAN'T KNOW WHAT to fix unless you know what's going on behind the scenes. Perhaps you have high blood pressure or stress is overwhelming you. Maybe some of your vitamin or other nutritional levels are low or, while working from home, you ate your emotions and gained unwanted weight. Perhaps you're on the verge of developing diabetes and existing treatments aren't working anymore.

Whatever your motivation for improving your health, the first step is getting to know yourself. Week 1 determines your baselines because you need to know where you stand in order to develop a plan. This first week helps you gather data about yourself—which tests you need and why—but you also will answer some tough questions, such as: Do you like your boss? Working for someone you hate can destroy your mental health, and an important part of the Immunity Solution Protocol consists of identifying what isn't working, whether physical or social. Lots of genetic and lifestyle factors play a huge role in how you feel. That's why it's so important to have an accurate assessment of your health status by looking at the whole picture of you. I provide the questions, and you need to answer them honestly. Fibbing shortchanges only you. Remember, your health is in your hands. If you've read this far, you have demonstrated a vested interest in changing the course of your health, so stay the course.

As you get to know yourself better and note your observations, you're preparing for Week 2, when you'll create a personal health book to track your stats. That book will become an invaluable tool that contains many snapshots of your health—like an animated flipbook—and can make conversations with healthcare providers much more effective. The self-exams, tests, and tips in this program don't replace a professional physical at the doctor's office, but they can help you understand when something might require medical attention. You also can perform these quick self-exams at home, between appointments, but remember that they supplement rather than replace proper professional care. If you have any kind of difficulty or disability that makes performing any of the following self-exams difficult, enlist the help of a trusted family member or friend.

BEFORE YOU BEGIN: HOW ARE YOU DOING?

How old do you feel? Some people spend a lifetime feeling ill, thinking it's normal to feel bad, but it isn't. In this first step, ask yourself the following questions:

- How old do I feel?
- Do I enjoy my life?
- When was the last time I felt fantastic?
- Do I feel joy when I wake every morning?
- Did I feel bloated or gassy over the past week?
- When was the last time I was sick?
- When was the last time I saw the doctor?
- What did my doctor tell me I had to do to improve my health?
- Am I following that directive?

- Does my community embrace me?
- What am I passionate about?
- Does it feel like my body needs a reset?
- Can I improve anything today?
- Am I on the right track for a long life?
- What are my health goals?

Answering these questions might trigger a range of emotions, so take it slow and do it over several days, if necessary. Don't be afraid to be honest, but be kind to yourself. Self-criticism can be as important as self-acceptance, but being gentle to yourself will help you down the road to recovery. Your own circumstances, decisions, and actions are entirely your affair and no one else's. Make your health a judgment-free zone, especially in your own thoughts.

Remember, all of these tests should be performed on a regular basis to give you information about how your body is doing. They should not replace annual wellness checks with your primary care physician. As you do these exams at home, be sure to keep track of your results so that you can spot any positive or negative patterns— before the latter become problems.

DAY 1: HOW'S YOUR SMILE?

For most of us, poor health creeps up when we're not paying attention. Research shows that, when you stop taking care of yourself, you stop looking in the mirror. Maybe you're avoiding what you don't want to face. Whatever the reason, it's time to take a look again because your life is worth it.

One day you're a happy toddler running around your home, and in the blink of an eye you become an adult with a list of prescriptions as long as your arm. Body parts ache that never hurt before, cuts take twice as long to heal, and the face in the mirror no longer smiles back. Even if physically you're a strong person, life some-times can get you down and make you feel exhausted.

Happy facial expressions—grin, smile, smirk—have a feel-good impact, but we smile less as we age. According to studies, young people smile 400 times per day on average, compared to just 20 times per day for the average adult.[80] Smiling not only improves your mood, but it also aids in the release of neurotransmitters that have several health benefits. Smiling is also contagious. It activates brain neurons that fire a synchronizing feature. One grin can cause others around you to smile as well. A wide range of conditions start in the mouth, but first let's see your smile because protecting that will help you protect other parts of your body.

Step 1: Smile in a Mirror

From cavities to oral cancer, oral health accurately reflects a healthy immune system and overall health. Brush your teeth at least twice a day, floss regularly, visit the dentist every 6 months, and check your mouth regularly.

Step 2: Check Your Gums and Teeth

Gum disease usually starts as gingivitis, an inflammation of the gums stemming from bacteria-rich plaque accumulating between your teeth, but that inflammation can lead to periodontitis, a con-dition in which the inner layer of the gums and bones pull away from the teeth and form pockets. These small spaces can collect even more bacteria that the immune system then tries to fight. In advanced periodontitis, the bone holding the teeth in place decays, and teeth become loose and often fall out. This infection can spread throughout your body and affect other major organs. You can reverse both gingivitis and periodontitis if you catch them early.

Your dentist does a basic oral health check every time you visit, but you can do it, too. Open wide and run a clean finger around the inside, feeling your gums and teeth as well as under your tongue. Check for any abnormalities. In this mouth check, you also are looking for signs of cancer. If you notice any changes in the shape or feel of your tongue, mouth, cheeks, or throat, notify your dentist and healthcare provider immediately.

Between dental visits, you can perform a more thorough oral health self-examination in a few easy steps:

1. Wash your hands with plain soap and cold water.
2. Remove any oral appliances, such as orthodontic devices, retainers, or dentures.
3. Along the sides and front of the neck, feel for tenderness or lumps.
4. Apply the same technique to the outside of your jaw.
5. Facing a mirror for the rest of the exam, pull your upper lip up and examine the underside of your lip and gums for sores or color changes.
6. Repeat with your lower lip.
7. With your fingers, pull out one of your cheeks and look inside your mouth for color changes such as red, white, or dark patches.
8. To feel for lumps, place your index finger on the inside of your cheek and your thumb on the outside.
9. Repeat on the opposite cheek.
10. With a clean gauze pad or folded paper towel, grasp your tongue, lift it up and side to side, and look for swellings or changes in color. Examine the top, back, and sides.
11. Touch your tongue to the roof of your mouth. Look at the underside and the floor of your mouth, checking for color shifts.
12. Feel for any unusual bumps, swelling, or tenderness with

one finger inside your mouth and one finger on the outside corresponding to the same place.

13. Repeat this exam several times per year.

Tell your dentist and physician right away if you notice any of the following:

- a mouth sore that bleeds profusely or doesn't heal
- a lump or thick spot in your cheek that your tongue can feel
- a white or red patch on the gums, tongue, or other part of your mouth
- persistent sore throat or sensation that something is stuck in your throat
- difficulty chewing or swallowing food
- difficulty moving your tongue or jaw
- numbness in your tongue or mouth
- swelling of the upper or lower jaw that causes oral appliances to fit incorrectly or causes pain
- sudden sensitivity in your teeth
- bad breath that doesn't go away
- jaw pain or lockjaw
- cracked or broken teeth
- sudden changes in how your teeth bite together

DAY 2: HOW'S YOUR SKIN?

For your immune system, your skin is one of your most important organs. Healthy skin doesn't come just from genetics. Your daily habits affect what you see in the mirror. Regular exposure to natural sunlight ensures that you obtain adequate vitamin D in the most effective way.

Step 1: 10–30 Minutes of Sunshine

Less than half an hour of sun exposure is completely safe and necessary to help the cells in your skin synthesize that light into vitamin D. Get 10 to 30 minutes of early morning or midday sunlight every day to keep your skin looking healthy and to boost your overall well-being. Even if the dead of winter has only a sliver of sunlight, chase it. People with darker skin may require more sunlight to obtain the appropriate levels of vitamin D.

If you get more sun exposure than necessary, such as in the yard, walking or hiking, or at the beach or pool, apply a mineral-based sunscreen to protect your skin from harmful UV rays. Sunscreen ingredients vary widely. Always read the labels and stay up to date on FDA recalls to ensure that the product you're using won't damage your health. Your sunscreen creates a barrier between you and long-term DNA damage to your skin, so it pays to buy a quality product that's safe for you, your immune system, and the environment. Choose one without cancer-causing chemicals or propellants in it. Sunscreens for babies or children are a good bet for the whole family. If you're swimming in the ocean, look for reef-safe brands that don't harm sea life.

Step 2: Look at Your Skin

According to current research, one in five Americans will develop skin cancer. It can affect anyone, regardless of skin tone, but it's highly treatable if detected early. If you can, see a dermatologist or skin specialist every other year or so. In between those visits, regularly perform this skin self-exam at home, which, if you haven't already, will help you become familiar with the typical appearance and feel of any birthmarks, moles, skin tags, sunspots, warts, and other features and help you look for skin cancers, such as melanoma.

ABCDE
(the first signs of a melanoma)

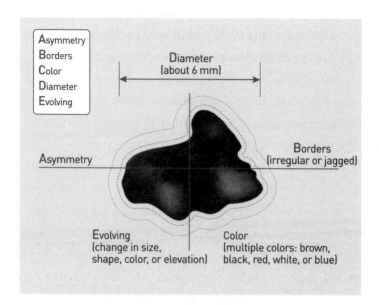

Asymmetry
Borders
Color
Diameter
Evolving

Diameter
(about 6 mm)

Asymmetry

Borders
(irregular or jagged)

Evolving
(change in size,
shape, color, or elevation)

Color
(multiple colors: brown,
black, red, white, or blue)

1. After a shower or bath, stand in a room with plenty of natural light, in front of a full-length mirror and using a handheld mirror.

2. Take off all clothing and jewelry.

3. Check your entire body from front to back.

4. Raise each arm and examine your right and left sides.

5. Look at the upper side of your arms and palms.

6. Bend your elbows and check the underside of your forearms and upper arms.

7. With the hand mirror, examine your armpits.

8. Look at your legs, the tops of your feet, and the spaces between your toes.

9. Turn around and check the backs of your legs and heels. Lift your feet and examine the spaces between your toes and the soles of your feet.

10. With the hand mirror, look at your neck and scalp, both front and back. Part your hair in areas where you may have more sun exposure.

11. Use a hand mirror to check your back and buttocks.

12. Repeat this exam several times per year.

Tell your skin specialist immediately if you notice any of the following:

- a change in the size, shape, or color of a mole
- a mole that looks different from your other moles
- a birthmark that has changed
- a new spot that hurts, itches, or bleeds
- a new, darker, red, or flaky patch of skin
- a patch of skin that feels or looks raised
- a patch of skin that feels reddish, warm, or inflamed
- a firm flesh-colored bump
- a sore that doesn't heal

If you notice anything unusual, take a picture and send it to your doctor. It might be harmless, such as a cherry angioma or a skin-tag, or it might be something serious. Your healthcare provider will tell you whether there's cause for concern, and having the picture will allow you to track when the condition first appeared and if it changes in the future.

DAY 3: HOW'S YOUR BELLY?

No one likes to talk about belly fat, but the conversation can save your life. It's not about whether you meet arbitrary beauty standards. It's about your health. You might have accepted an increase in your weight and fat deposits as a product of chronic stress or as an inevitable fact of aging. But as your waistline grows, so do your health risks. Belly fat produces hormones that increase health risks for a wide range of diseases. And it doesn't stop at the surface. Visceral fat, which surrounds your internal organs, adds to that pooch that many of us develop. Compared with the subcutaneous kind, visceral fat correlates with far more serious health issues, such as impaired immunity, heart disease, type 2 diabetes, and high blood pressure.

For most people, weight management typically begins with waist management, so let's see where you stand.

Step 1: Measure Your Waist

To perform a belly fat measurement, follow these steps:

1. Standing in front of a full-length mirror, remove your clothes and any accessories.
2. At belly button level, wrap a loose tape measure around your waist. Make sure it's not too tight or too loose.
3. Exhale normally but don't suck in your stomach. Note the number.
4. Repeat this test monthly.

Women should have a waist circumference of 35 inches or fewer. For men, that number is 40 inches or fewer. Always perform this self-exam under the same conditions, such as in the morning, after going to the bathroom but before breakfast. If your number is higher than the recommended measurement, talk to your doctor about what you can do to manage your weight.

Step 2: Commit to Improving Your Habits

If your waistline or overall health isn't where you want it to be, now's the time to implement change. You're reading this book, so you already have committed to learning more about being healthy.

This program eases you into creating habits that are good for your health. If some of the steps seem difficult, go back to the questions you answered before you began the protocol. Use those answers to motivate yourself and commit to living better and longer.

DAY 4: HOW'S YOUR HEART?

Heart disease is the leading cause of death for men and women. On average, heart attacks cut 15 years off people's lives. According to the CDC, as many as 89 percent of sudden cardiac events occur in men.[81] People who have had a heart attack are four to six times more likely to die suddenly. The AHA recommends taking your pulse regularly to monitor your heart's health. Smartwatches can do it automatically for you. Recent generations of the Apple Watch also perform a blood oxygen test and can run a mini echocardiogram. You can configure most smartwatches to alert you if your heart rate strays beyond a chosen number of beats per minute (BPM).

Step 1: Check Your Pulse

Here's how to perform a quick heart-health test without a device.

1. Find a comfortable resting position, sitting or lying down. Place the first two fingers of one hand on the base of the wrist, just before the point where it meets your hand. If you can't detect your pulse at your wrist, try your jugular vein, which runs up the side of your neck, just below the curve of the right side of your jaw.
2. Set a timer or stopwatch for 60 seconds. Measure your pulse by counting the number of beats you feel in 60 seconds.
3. Repeat this exam once a month.

To check your heart rate using a smartwatch, open the heart rate app, which, if you wear it regularly, can provide your average heart rate when resting, walking, and working out, giving you an even more thorough understanding of your measurements.

At rest, your heart rate should fall between 60 and 80 BPM. A resting rate more than 80 BPM could indicate cardiovascular problems, in which case tell your physician right away.

Step 2: Check Your Blood Pressure

According to the AHA, high blood pressure can result in heart attack, heart failure, stroke, kidney failure, and other health complications. Many drug stores or pharmacies have a dedicated blood pressure testing machine, or you can buy a blood pressure monitor. To measure your blood pressure effectively, follow these steps:

1. If you take blood pressure medication, measure your blood pressure before you take your medication.
2. Avoid caffeine, nicotine, and other stimulants for at least 30 minutes before you measure your blood pressure. Also wait at least 30 minutes after eating.
3. Too much liquid in the body can put pressure on your organs and raise your blood pressure, so empty your bladder beforehand.
4. Find a quiet space where you can sit comfortably without distraction.
5. For the duration of the test, keep your legs uncrossed and avoid conversations and watching TV or other screens.
6. Put the cuff on snugly, but not too tight.
7. Rest comfortably for 5 minutes.
8. Press the button on the monitor and remain relaxed and still.
9. Record your measurements when finished.

10. Spacing them 1 minute apart, take one or two more measurements and average the numbers.

11. Repeat this exam monthly.

This test will give you two numbers, systolic (maximum pressure during one heartbeat) and diastolic (minimum pressure between two heartbeats). The AHA has identified the following five key blood pressure ranges:

< 120 / 80, normal

Stick with your existing heart-healthy habits, such as following a balanced diet and getting regular exercise.

120–129 / < 80, elevated

People with elevated blood pressure probably will develop high blood pressure unless they take steps to control the situation.

130–139 / 80–89, hypertension stage 1

For these ranges, a doctor probably will prescribe lifestyle changes and may consider medication, depending on risk factors for cardio-vascular disease, such as heart attack or stroke.

> 140 / 90, hypertension stage 2

At this range, your healthcare provider probably will prescribe both medication and lifestyle changes.

> 180 / 120, hypertensive crisis

These numbers require immediate medical attention. To rule out a measurement error, wait calmly for 5 minutes and test again. If the reading remains this high or if you're experiencing chest pain, shortness of breath, back pain, numbness or weakness, or changes in vision or speaking, call immediately for emergency help.

DAY 5: HOW ARE YOUR PRIVATE PARTS?

Even if you're shy or squeamish about your body, you need to take care of *all* of it, including your private parts. Ask your healthcare provider for basic screenings for sexually transmitted infections and diseases and keep a regular eye on your genitals and chest.

Breast Self-Exam

This exam can help you understand how your breasts should look and feel, and breast cancer is one of the few cancers that you can detect early and at home. The technique doesn't always offer a reliable way to detect breast cancer—as compared to a mammogram, which, if you have certain risk factors, you should have annually—but many women report that a lump discovered on their own was the first sign of disease. If you discover a lump, don't panic. The majority of changes or lumps discovered during a self-exam are benign, but some changes can indicate more serious issues.

Hormone levels fluctuate each month during the menstrual cycle, which causes changes in breast tissue. When your period starts, the normal swelling of your breasts begins to decrease. If you're menstruating, choose a time in your cycle when your breasts feel least tender. The best time to perform a self-exam for breast awareness is usually the week after your period ends.

Before doing the following exam at home, ask your gynecologist, physician, or a nurse for a demonstration. A breast self-exam has two parts: a visual check and a manual check. When doing any kind of self-exam, use the pads of your fingers, not the tips, so you can feel more tissue more effectively. Take your time. Don't rush. Be gentle.

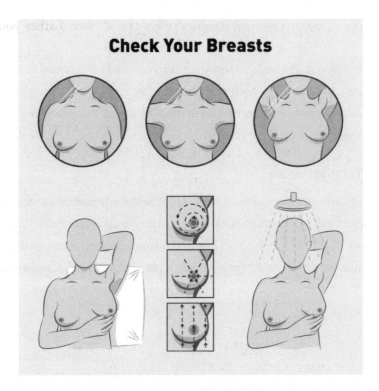

Check Your Breasts

1. Stand in front of a mirror without wearing a top or bra.

2. Face forward, arms at your sides. Check for any changes in your skin.

3. Examine for any puckering, dimpling, or changes in size, shape, or symmetry.

4. Note whether your nipples are turned in or inverted.

5. Press your hands to your hips and look at your breasts.

6. Raise your arms overhead, palms pressed together, and check your breasts again.

7. Lift one breast at a time to see whether the ridges along the bottom look symmetrical or unusual.

8. For the manual part of the exam, lie down on a bed or other flat surface. When you're lying down, your breast tissue spreads, making it thinner and easier to feel. You

also can do a manual exam in the shower. Lather your fingers and breasts with soap to help your fingers glide more smoothly over your skin.

9. Feel for any lumps or changes.
10. Repeat this exam once a month.

Many women notice lumps or changes in their breasts, which commonly occur at various times during the menstrual cycle. Breasts can have a variety of sensations, depending on which part you're feeling. For example, a normal firm ridge runs along the bottom of each breast. As you age, your breasts will change in appearance and feel. Men can develop analogous chest cancers, so the above exam can help everyone.

Tell your doctor if you notice any of the following:

- hard lumps
- a knot near your underarm
- changes in how your breasts look or feel
- thickening or swelling
- dimples, puckers, bulges, or ridges on the skin
- recent nipple inversion (turning inward)
- redness or warmth
- swelling or pain
- itchiness of the breast
- sores or rashes
- bloody nipple discharge

A breast self-exam supplements but doesn't replace a clinical breast exam or screening mammogram.

Testicular Self-Exam

This exam can help you understand how your testicles should look and feel. Changes can indicate a common benign condition, such as an infection or cyst, or more serious issues. When doing any kind of

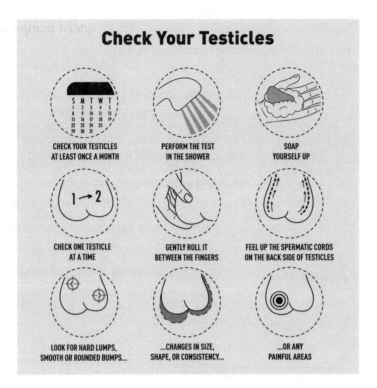

self-exam, use the pads of your fingers, not the tips, so you can feel more tissue more effectively. Take your time. Don't rush. Be gentle.

1. Take a warm bath or shower, which relaxes the scrotum, making it easier to check for anything unusual.
2. Standing in front of a mirror, hold your penis out of the way and examine the skin of the scrotum.
3. Using both hands, place your index and middle fingers under one testicle and your thumbs on top. Look at each testicle separately.
4. Between your thumbs and fingers, gently roll each testicle, one at a time. Check for any abnormalities or signs of swelling.

5.   Examine for any hard lumps, smooth rounded bumps, or changes in size, shape, or consistency.

Not every lump or bump is cause for worry. While performing this self-exam, you may notice bumps on the skin of your scrotum, which often result from ingrown hairs, rashes, or other skin issues. You may notice a soft, ropy cord, which is the epididymis, a normal part of the scrotum. It extends upward from the top rear of each testicle.

Tell your physician or urologist if you notice any of the following:

- lumps
- pain
- changes since your last self-exam
- swelling
- fluid around your testicles
- unusual redness or warmth

DAY 6: ARE YOU STRESSED OUT?

According to the National Institute of Mental Health, stress is a natural, healthy response. At some point in our lives, as a result of various situations, we all experience significant levels of it. But persistent, chronic stress can damage your health and requires medical attention. Always feeling overwhelmed, rushed for time, or like you're walking on eggshells is bad for you. You deserve to be happy, and the near-constant flow of stress hormones, especially cortisol, can age you more quickly and make your body more susceptible to sickness. This questionnaire will help determine whether you have excessive stress in your life.

Step 1: Determine Your Stress Level

QUESTION	ANSWER	
Do you feel exhausted all the time?	YES	NO
Do you have difficulty sleeping more than one night a week?	YES	NO
Do you have a hard time relaxing?	YES	NO
Do you feel "attached" to your phone?	YES	NO
Do you experience brain fog more than one day a week?	YES	NO
Have you lost your temper in the last week?	YES	NO
Have you shouted at your phone in the last week?	YES	NO
Have you shouted at another person in the last week?	YES	NO
Do you frequently feel angry at the end of the day?	YES	NO
Do you often argue about minor things?	YES	NO
Do you feel that you never have time for yourself?	YES	NO
Do others tell you that you need a break?	YES	NO
Do you feel that you never have downtime?	YES	NO
Do you just want to be left alone?	YES	NO
Do you sometimes wish that you could disappear?	YES	NO
TOTAL NUMBER		

Each of us has bad experiences and days, and we all experience some of the symptoms above from time to time. But if you responded "yes" to two or more of these questions and feel this way on a regular basis, you are stressed! That's not good for your immune system or your overall health. You may be underestimating your ability to cope with stress in your daily life. In Week 6, we delve into coping strategies for calming mind and body.

DAY 7: HOW ARE YOUR ENERGY LEVELS?

Lots of people feel like they're running on fumes. Even if they don't feel depleted, exhaustion can manifest in a variety of ways. Even if they get enough sleep each night, some people feel chronically exhausted. Others begin the day with plenty of power and vitality but quickly run out of steam. Persistent feelings of malaise or listlessness, coupled with frequently feeling physically weak, indifferent, or emotionally vulnerable, indicate a more serious underlying problem.

We'll talk about exercise later in the program, but this isn't about strength or speed. It's about stamina, several different fitness components that combine into endurance. When days run long or contain stressful situations, stamina can mean the difference between feeling depleted and being able to rebound quickly and move on to the next thing.

Step 1: Check Your Stamina

Ask yourself the following questions:

- Can you run quickly over longer distances? How fast and how far?
- Can you lift heavier weights for a high number of repetitions? How much and how many reps?

- Can you hike for a decent period of time? How long?
- Do you feel physically fit?
- Could you successfully handle a high-stress, long-hours job?
- Does your mental strength hold throughout the day?

Many supercentenarians that I researched for this book remained active physically and mentally long into old age. That combination of living a healthy lifestyle and staying active gives them stamina. They can endure whatever comes their way and bounce back when they suffer setbacks.

Week 2.

TRACK YOUR HEALTH

YOUR DOCTOR HAS A MEDICAL CHART FOR YOU THAT COMPILES ALL AVAILable data about your health. Decades ago, these charts started on paper, but advancements in technology have transformed them. From paper to megabytes, digital records have added convenience but also the potential for security breaches. As medical records cross platforms, they allow doctors in different specialties and offices to access your information as needed. Today, it's more critical than ever that none of your information be incomplete or wrong.

Between doctor visits, a health journal can fill the gaps. You are your own best advocate, so never give all knowledge or control of your health to someone else. Seeing at a glance when you received your most recent flu shot, when your seasonal allergies flare up, how your menstrual cycle fluctuates, or when a bad night's sleep made you feel like a wreck can help you make better decisions about how to live your life. That information also can help you have more effective conversations with your health professionals.

In a perfect world, you'd have one big chart from the day you were born and update it every time your health or life patterns changed.

That technology isn't possible yet, but a health journal can do much the same thing. According to a recent study, patients with heart failure who kept a health journal had a higher chance of survival.

Most people think of the human brain as a storage device, but in practice it's better at processing information than storing it. Don't rely on your memory. Write the data down. Doing so will free some of your mental reserves, reduce worry, and help you remember the important stuff when you speak with your healthcare providers. Your health journal also puts you in the driver's seat. Seeing your symptoms in writing on a page can help you understand them better and give you a sense of control if something goes wrong. This journal will give you autonomy over your body and any treatment plans. You also don't have to worry about forgetting to mention something when you talk to your doctor. The typical medical visit lasts fewer than 15 minutes, which makes it easy to feel rushed or forget something.

You can create one on paper or digitally by making tagged notes in your phone's calendar or using a specific health app. You can use your phone to track what you eat, how many steps you take each day, and what exercise you do, and you can record all of that on paper, too. I prefer a health journal on paper because that format makes it easy to flip through and see patterns or results. In this section, you'll receive field-tested advice about what you should track, when you should track it, and what information isn't worth the effort.

DAYS 1 TO 3: CREATE A HEALTH JOURNAL

This record doesn't have to contain solely medical information. It's your book, so add whatever you find important, from how you feel in general to the details of work stress. But remember that your emotional health and mental health connect to your physical health, so pay attention to all of it.

It can be as simple or as complex as you like, but include as much health information as possible. Before you start, you may want to contact your doctor's office for a copy of your medical records. That's a great time to double-check that all your health-care providers have the same information. A good question always to keep in mind: "Should my doctor know about this?" If so, write it down. Start fresh, add as much information as possible, remain consistent, and keep it accurate. If you ate 10 cookies after lunch but wrote down only 2, that defeats the purpose of the book. Identify day-to-day habits, foods, liquids, and products. Note everything you eat, drink, consume, touch, and use in a 24-hour period. Repeat the process for 4 more days, excluding the weekend. Why? We often behave differently on weekends, and we want to focus only on daily habits.

Not everything's worth tracking, though. If you feel good, you don't need to note how many times you go to the toilet in a day. If you have diarrhea regularly, however, your doctor should know, and details can help. You already know to brush your teeth and floss daily, so no need to focus on those metrics, either—unless you're not good at maintaining those good habits and need to establish baselines. In general, don't worry about every single data point available on an app or health-keeping device. That level of scrutiny can make you feel anxious, overwhelmed, or discouraged, which isn't helpful.

Instead, focus on the big-picture items that matter most. Here, at a minimum, is what your health journal should contain.

Emergency Information

Whom should your family or healthcare providers call if you have any urgent health issues? What's your insurance information? What are the names and numbers of your doctors? What allergies do you have? Do you have any advanced life directives, such as a do-not-resuscitate order? Have you selected a loved one as your healthcare proxy? In an emergency, do you need someone to watch your pet, tell your boss or landlord, or take care of your plants?

Health History

What's your family health history, on both your maternal and paternal sides? Are there any genetic conditions your doctor should know about? Has anything changed with a close relative? When was your last surgery? When was your last physical? How did it go? Was there a follow-up? Have you solved that health issue? Have you developed any new symptoms?

Vaccination History

Gather all of your vaccination records and keep them in a secure place that you'll remember, then write down in your health journal what vaccines you had and when. If you can't find your vax records, ask if your doctor has them on file and ask for a copy. Also ask if you need any boosters, including for various strains of hepatitis. Consider the following vaccines.

Everyone who is able should have a COVID vaccine and boosters within the time frames recommended by the manufacturers (Pfizer-BioNTech, Moderna, Johnson & Johnson, AstraZeneca). You can mix and match them for increased coverage. Everyone can get an annual influenza vaccine, but adults over age 50 absolutely should. As all viruses do, the flu virus mutates, so last year's vaccine may not work against this year's predominant strain. You can receive a flu shot and COVID vaccine or booster at the same time. For people over 65, a high-dose influenza vaccine, also called an adjuvanted flu shot, contains four times the antigens as the standard vaccine and an additional ingredient that promotes a better immune response. Middle-aged people with existing conditions, especially asthma, diabetes, kidney disease, heart disease or stroke, lung disease, liver disorders, weakened immune systems, obesity, endocrine disorders, or metabolic disorders, are more likely to develop serious flu complications, so if you fall into any of those categories, get a flu shot every year.

If you're 50 or older, get a pneumonia and a shingles vaccine to keep your immune system up to date. For most adults, a single shot of the pneumonia vaccine is sufficient. Those with a cochlear implant or a cerebrospinal fluid leak require two shots spaced 8 weeks apart. Anyone age 65 or older or who has a chronic medical condition, such as smoking, alcoholism, lung disease, liver disease, or heart disease, should get the pneumonia shot, which typically lasts 10 years. To prevent shingles—a painful, blistering rash that can cause nerve pain for several months or longer in a third of people—get the Shingrix vaccine, which consists of two shots separated by 2 to 3 months.

If you haven't been vaccinated in the last 5 years against tetanus, diphtheria, or pertussis, you need a booster shot every 10 years or after a puncture wound. If unvaccinated, tetanus, a potentially fatal bacterial infection, has no cure. Diphtheria affects the heart, kidneys, lungs, and nervous system, particularly in older people. Pertussis, also called whooping cough, can prove particularly dangerous for infants and young children. The DTP vaccine protects against all three. People aged 65 and older should take the Boostrix version.

Current Medication List

Research shows that, because different healthcare providers didn't communicate properly, patients often are overprescribed or mix contraindicated medications. Write down all the medications you take, along with current dosages and directions. Note why you take them and whether you need to take them forever. If any of them has caused any adverse reactions in the past, detail the circumstances. Side effects and adverse reactions are possible with any medication, so ask your physician whether all of your medications are safe to take with one another *and* with the supplements that you take.

Current Supplement List

You have ready access to all kinds of vitamins, minerals, sleep aids, herbal remedies, CBD, and in some places THC and other psychoactive plants and drugs. Taken together or separately, what you consume affects your health and well-being in one way or another. A cancer patient once told me he took "a couple of vitamins" every day. When I asked him to show me, he presented 23 bottles! As with your medications, keep track of all the supplements you take, along with dosages and directions. Note why you take them and whether you plan on taking them forever. Tell your doctor because some supplements can interfere with medication, particularly Saint-John's-wort and activated charcoal. They also can cause side effects, as was the case with a friend who turned out to have an allergy to OTC sleep aids.

What You Eat Regularly

Keep tabs on the types, quantities, and calories of food you're eating. Note if you had a reaction to a particular food. Also note what you drink, including water, caffeinated beverages, sugary drinks, or alcohol.

In addition to the health reasons that we already have discussed, you should tell your healthcare providers about what you consume because some foods and liquids can cause food-drug interactions. Other foods can prevent certain medicines from working or improve, worsen, or create new medicinal side effects. Drugs can change the way your body uses food, too. Green, leafy vegetables, high in vitamin K, can decrease how well aspirin thins the blood. Grapefruit juice alters the way the body absorbs cholesterol-lowering drugs, such as Lipitor, and calcium channel blockers. Dairy products decrease the absorption of antibiotics.

Alcohol Consumption

As you learned in the chapter on the power of habits, drinking little to no alcohol is the healthiest way to go because it can have a profound effect on the body. But always be honest with your doctor about how much and how often you drink. One unit equals 10 milliliters or 8 grams of pure alcohol, which is roughly how much exists in one 8-ounce serving of beer, one 5-ounce serving of wine, or one 1½-ounce serving of liquor. Do the math and don't fib. Your doctor's trying to help you live a good, long life. All your care providers need accurate information to do that.

Alcohol prolongs the effects of injectable insulin and oral diabetic pills, which can lead to low blood sugar. Never take any pain reliever containing acetaminophen with or after alcohol because the combination has a higher chance of causing severe liver damage. Also avoid antihistamines, such as Benadryl, with alcohol because they increase drowsiness.

Environmental Items

List everything that goes into or touches your body, which will help you and your doctor spot potential toxins or triggers. Note:

- personal care products, such as cotton swabs, tampons, cotton balls, bandages;
- hygiene items, including soaps, shampoos, body butters, nose cleaners, douche items, perfumes, colognes;
- skin care products, such as cleansers, moisturizers, sunscreens;

- oral care items, including toothpaste, mouthwash, dental floss;
- OTC drugs, such as pain relievers, allergy pills, antacids, laxatives;
- accessories, including earrings, bracelets, glasses, and watches, because some metals can cause reactions.

How You're Feeling

It may seem like a simple question, but noticing the last time you felt good can provide helpful information. Sometimes simple questions have complex answers. For instance, a stomachache that lasts a day might have come from eating something bad. A stomachache for several days could be a sign of something more serious. Being precise with your doctor—"I started having these symptoms 6 days ago"—helps determine whether something is serious.

Good Days

A grateful heart beats better. In addition to noting how you feel physically, also record brief notes about your mental health. Doing that can help you find something good that happened in a given time frame, even if it's a minor moment.

DAYS 4 TO 6: TRACK YOUR HABITS

Once you complete or update your health journal, it's time to look more closely at some of your daily habits. Answer these questions to identify what you might need to improve or what may be harming your immunity.

- Do you drink tap water at home, work, or elsewhere?
- On a scale of 0–5 (0 is awful, 5 is awesome), how well did you sleep?

- How many times did you brush your teeth?
- Did you do laundry or clean the kitchen or bathroom?
- Did you touch any industrial materials
  or anyone that works with them?
- Did you smoke, vape, or use any other nicotine products?
- What physical activity did you do today?
- On the same 0–5 scale, how do you feel?

If you didn't know your age, how old would you say you are? The answer to that question says quite a bit about your age. How you feel reflects how well your systems, organs, and cells are running. Tracking the answers to these questions can help you identify immunity-harming culprits in your food, water, or household items. But doing this work requires commitment and bold self-awareness. No one enjoys taking notes all the time, but a complete picture of your health will give you invaluable information, itself a powerful and life-changing tool. Knowledge allows you to take action and have control of your health.

With this exercise, you're looking for keys to improve daily habits to get the most from your immune system. Listing those habits helps you see areas for improvement. When you wake up, do you brush your teeth right away? That's a habit. After lunch, do you smoke a cigarette every day? That's another habit. Do you always eat everything on your plate, even if you're full? Do you watch TV every night after dinner? Do you drink a glass of water before going to bed? All habits. Identifying them helps you ditch any that no longer serve your health. If keeping this journal helps you realize that you eat or drink your feelings, you've won the first battle. You can make necessary changes because now you know the problem.

You also can use your journal as a form of diary. It can help you discover inner feelings and thoughts and connect the dots between your health and your life. Use it to write down aspirations, plans, and goals. Record vulnerabilities, fears, and other emotions that affect your health. If you like, you can divide the book into two sections: a private part for your eyes only and one for your health professionals. Don't withhold important medical information from them, but you also don't have tell them absolutely everything happening in your head. It's all about identifying and sharing the right information so you can build the healthiest possible life.

It takes 21 days to develop a new habit. Make today Day 1 with your health journal.

DAY 7: CHECK YOUR HABITS

One of the most common mistakes that people make regarding their health is underestimating the influence of what they do every day. How you wake up, when you eat your first meal, the time you go to bed—all of it serves as the blueprint for your internal operating system. Your brain wants to do what it knows how to do best *all the time*, which means it brings you back to the same actions, tasks, or thoughts over and over again—even if they're bad for you. That's why many of us become trapped in cycles of bad habits and behaviors.

It can prove difficult to maintain good changes and habits over the long haul. For example, smokers often drink coffee, another stimulant, while smoking. They frequently fail to quit smoking because their brains encounter the caffeine and then expect the nicotine to follow. That action-reaction cycle can activate cravings and create trouble. After 7 days, review everything you've written in your health journal. Determine what you want to stop, what's important to you, and what you cannot live without. Identifying what you do when and why is a critical step on your health journey.

Consider this next exercise an objective investigation of your health. Put yourself in the shoes of a private investigator looking for clues.

Step 1: Identify Every Habit

Answer the following questions:

- What time do you wake up?
- Do you use an alarm to wake up?
- Do you check your phone as soon as you wake up?
- Do you check the news, email, or social media as soon as you grab your phone?
- Do you ever wake up thinking that you need to change your life?
- If you woke up an hour earlier than usual, what would you do with that time?
- Do you meditate or focus on a moment of calm before starting your day?
- Do you eat real, whole foods for the most part?
- How much of your food needs refrigeration?
- How much of your food comes from packages?
- In the past month, have you gained, maintained, or lost weight?
- When was the last time you binge-ate?
- Do you overeat when stressed?
- When was the last time you fasted?
- What's your favorite part of your day and why?
- Do you have a set routine for the day? For bedtime?
- Do you meditate or focus on a moment of calm before ending your day?
- Are your habits leading you toward better health or away from it? How?
- What would it take to improve your daily routines?

Week 3.

EAT BETTER

WITH EASY-TO-FOLLOW GUIDANCE, YOU CAN START EATING HEALTHIER TODAY and for the next 3 weeks without breaking the bank. Based on research validated for decades, this section will give you a basic understanding of eating for better health. You'll discover new foods, new habits, and new ideas about eating. You also will learn how your new eating habits can lead to increased longevity, beginning a 21-day reset with the Immunity Solution Diet and concluding with a maintenance plan. During these 21 days, you must abstain from alcohol, tobacco, heavy-metal exposure, and ultraprocessed foods. That's the bad news. The good news is that what you can eat tastes delicious, the diet has no calorie restrictions, and you might lose some weight.

I'll forewarn you: The Immunity Solution Diet runs a little on the strict side. You're eliminating foods that can cause immunological reactions. But don't let that deter you. This critical phase will provide your body with a much-needed opportunity for your defense mechanisms to take a breather and reset. This elimination plan excludes foods that researchers believe commonly trigger unfavorable reactions, also called food intolerances. Most of us picture food reactions like anaphylaxis with peanuts. But your body can react to foods in other, slower ways that might be affecting your immune system. Clinical experience has identified an exclusion diet as one of the most effective techniques for identifying these triggers. It's also safe, provided that you maintain good nutrient variety.

A variety of ingredients and compounds in packaged foods—such as additives, artificial colors, preservatives, and flavorings—can cause food intolerances and immune reactions in the body. You'll be eliminating particular foods for a period of 21 days, but you won't reintroduce them or challenge your body, as with traditional elimination diets. If your current diet is high in sugars, carbohydrates, and ultraprocessed junk, you may feel withdrawal symptoms. That reaction will tell you which foods are causing you to feel fatigued or unwell as well as which foods are making you age faster.

The human body digests, absorbs, and stores organic and naturally occurring products with high efficiency—but only if junk isn't getting in the way or undoing the benefits of the good foods you are ingesting. Even though the diet takes only 21 days, it has the potential to be life changing.

DAY 1: WHAT IT TAKES TO EAT HEALTHY

Immune disruptors lurk in a lot of foods and liquids that you probably consume right now, from lead in your water to preservatives in your favorite chips. These disruptors can damage healthy cells while evading detection by your immune cells. According to the National Institutes of Health, they can interfere with hormone interactions, destabilize beneficial gut bacteria, and in some cases induce life-threatening disorders. That's why people with immunological disorders and autoimmune diseases find this diet, which eliminates those disruptors entirely, extremely beneficial.

Many people have reported that, by following this program and adopting its healthy practices, they have lost weight and feel healthier. Weight loss isn't the objective, but it can be a happy side effect. The goal of the Immunity Solution Diet is to enhance your defense mechanisms and prevent health damage.

Step 1: Avoid Immune Disruptors

Many years of working in drug discovery as an immunologist and immunotherapy scientist have made it clear to me that bad dietary habits are harming people's immune systems. This diet will help people with specific immune disorders, but it also helps anyone interested in developing better eating habits. If you have frequent gastrointestinal issues, your body is trying to tell you that you're consuming something bad for you. One factor often can lead to gastrointestinal issues as well as immunological disorders. Sometimes a combination of factors is causing the problems.

The first step is identifying anything that you consume that contains or may contain pesticides, preservatives, heavy metals, and other toxins. You need to read the labels, know the sources of your produce and protein, and accept that you shouldn't ingest something made on a factory line and filled with ingredients you can't pronounce. This step is just about gathering information and thinking, though. Look at what you eat regularly and ask yourself if a nutritionist or doctor would tell you that it's healthy. If you know that something may have contributed to health problems in the past, try eliminating that (again) before making any dietary changes or adding supplements to your regimen.

Step 2: What's on Your Veggies?

Fresh vegetables and fruits provide lots of micronutrients and help you stay healthier. Some of them contain probiotic and even anti-inflammatory properties, but they also can contain harmful chemicals that counteract all those good benefits. Unless you source your food locally and during peak season, you probably are coming into contact with pesticides. Growers harvest regular veggies and fruits, imported from other countries, before they ripen fully to ensure that they don't decay before reaching the store. That means that they matured under the influence of pesticides. By the time you buy and eat them, the risks far outweigh the benefits.

According to recent studies, organic goods in America, which are subject to stringent restrictions, still may contain pesticide residues.[82] Research has revealed that pesticides and other chemical compounds have tainted up to 25 percent of organic produce before it even reaches store shelves. Organic foods may have lower amounts of pesticides, but all pesticides pose a serious hazard to your health and immune system, and you can't taste, smell, or see these dangerous chemicals. If you want to eat a salad for health reasons, follow the logic all the way through. Either know the source or test the food for biocides before eating it. If you can't do either, it's better not to eat it at all. If you find it difficult to exclude all crop vegetables from your diet, look for nearby farms or farmers' markets that sell organic veggies without pesticides.

Also invest in pesticide tests, readily available on the market, which can detect those potentially harmful chemicals. If it's in your food, it's probably in your bloodstream too.

DAY 2: WEIGHT LOSS STARTS IN THE GROCERY STORE

Contrary to popular belief and fitness marketing, exercise won't make you lose weight. It can suppress your appetite for a little while, which can help you manage your intake, but remember that your body craves homeostasis. The more you exercise, the more you'll want to eat. The type and amount of food you consume correlate directly with weight loss. If you need to drop some excess body fat, follow the next two steps.

Step 1: Three Secrets to Weight Loss

Don't Eat Breakfast

Your cortisol levels peak between 6 and 8 a.m., which means your body is ready to burn fat then. Start your day with 20 ounces of room-temperature water. You can have one espresso as well. To avoid caffeine anxiety, don't drink lots of brewed or iced coffee. Stick to one shot of espresso with no added creamers or sweeteners.

Eat Less

Try cutting your food consumption in half. Eat your first meal around 2 p.m., which gives your fasting body plenty of time to burn its own fat stores for fuel. Plate whatever you normally eat in the same way you always have but consume only half of it. Stop eating, acknowledge that you don't feel hungry anymore, and note how much food you're leaving behind. Refrigerate the remainder for lunch or dinner tomorrow. Having a visual of exactly how much you're eating will help you eat more mindfully in the future.

No Snacks

If you feel hungry, stressed, or bored, drink water or snack on some blueberries. No ultraprocessed snacks. If necessary, chew one stick of natural, sugar-free gum, but that's it.

Avoid nutritionless food to curb weight gain.

Step 2: Learn to Fast

For thousands of years, humans have used fasting for various reasons and in various forms. The Babylonians, Greeks (Stoics, Pythagoreans, Neoplatonists), and Romans all fasted. Today adherents of Zoroastrianism, Judaism, Christianity, and Islam all practice one version of it or another. If you found yourself on a deserted island and had to hunt for food and water, you certainly would lose weight. *Castaway*, starring Tom Hanks, excellently portrays this scenario. In modern Western civilization, we eat excessively because food is abundant and easy to obtain. You're not hunting for it on a deserted island. You can order from any restaurant or store and have that food delivered to your door in roughly 30 minutes.

Every 5 years, the USDA publishes *Dietary Guidelines for Americans*. It recommends women eat 1,600–2,400 calories per day and men 2,000–3,000 to maintain a healthy functioning body.[83] If we're lucky, we get about 80 years to live. Do you really want to count calories every day of that time? Calorie restriction is necessary for weight loss, and fasting can help you lose weight. An easy way to restrict your calorie intake, fasting jumpstarts your metabolism and makes the most of your body's natural processes.

One of the easiest and most effective ways to fast is to skip breakfast. I know it sounds hard. A heaping plate of buttermilk pancakes and bacon used to be one of my favorite morning dishes. But having a massive sugar rush first thing in the morning isn't healthy in the long run.

While you're starting your day, the cortisol in your body is telling your body to use its own fat as fuel. Your growth hormones are highest in the morning because you've been fasting overnight. Growth hormone has a lipolytic effect, meaning that it prefers to liberate fat from accumulated deposits and use that as fuel. This one-two punch gives your body more opportunities to burn fat while preserving muscle mass. The most effective way to sabotage this process is to eat as soon as you wake up.

All carbohydrates you consume convert to glucose and release into your bloodstream. Insulin, the storage hormone, removes glucose from the bloodstream. Insulin not only will do that, but it also will remove the free fatty acids generated earlier by cortisol. Losing weight becomes harder when that happens. Insulin's polar opposite is glucagon, a hormone that stimulates the release of glycogen (carbohydrates stored in our muscles) for the purpose of providing fuel. Insulin and glucagon have an inverse relationship, similar to the relationship between darkness and sunlight. When one of the two is absent, you get the other. As your blood sugar levels rise, insulin responds by putting glucagon into "hiding," which means your body can't burn those carbohydrates for fuel. Glucagon reappears only after the effects of glucose and insulin have faded. Glucagon also increases the release of growth hormone, which helps build muscle and slow aging, two more important reasons not to eat first thing in the morning.

Skipping breakfast uses those peak times for hormones to your advantage. Instead of eating breakfast, follow these steps in the morning.

- Don't reach for your phone: Blue light interferes with many of your body's mechanisms, and an overwhelming amount of information in the morning can derail your mindset, triggering anxiety and stress.
- Meditate in bed: Even just 5 minutes will help set the tone for your day.
- Optimize your brain flow: Neuromeditation with a brain device can help with neuromodulation, a targeted delivery of nerve activity. NeoRhythm targets specific parts of your brain to assist with achieving meditation goals by introducing low gamma waves of 34 hertz.

- Drink fresh, mineral-rich water: Staying hydrated helps you feel satisfied and keeps all of your systems running smoothly. Many Japanese people, one of the healthiest and slimmest populations, drink water immediately after waking.

- Have a shot of espresso: Get your coffee fix for the day with no creams or sweeteners. Just pure, concentrated coffee to get your brain and body ready to roll.

DAY 3: START THE IMMUNITY SOLUTION DIET

Supercentenarians (age 110+) live well-balanced lives and still enjoy some unhealthy habits, such as a glass of red wine or one cigarette a day. What's important is that they don't overindulge. The Immunity Solution Diet can feel a little restrictive, but if you like good food and wine, including cake and chocolate, you'll be able to eat some. Not always—and definitely not every day—but you won't completely lose what you truly enjoy.

The Immunity Solution Diet protects and empowers the immune system. A no-crops diet, it eliminates pesticides and other chemicals that can trigger or damage your defenses. It contains lots of meats while limiting exposure to toxins in other foods and drinks. At first glance, it may look like a carnivore diet because it relies heavily on real animal proteins, but the intent differs from trendy caveman regimens. It resets your immune system by feeding your cells exactly what they need. It's a low-carb, high-protein, anti-inflammatory diet that promotes good gut health. It allows your body to rebuild the immunity that a lifetime of exposure to chemicals, heavy metals, and poor choices has eroded. A healthy diet not only helps your kidneys, liver, and whole body recover, but it also helps you appreciate the joy of new foods.

Follow it for 21 days. If you smoke or vape, quit for these 3 weeks to give your lungs and heart a chance to repair themselves. You can't eat right and expect to feel healthy if you still inhale carcinogens. Kill that habit and look at others that you should put on hold during these 21 days. After that, you'll proceed to the maintenance phase (page 226).

But What About . . . ?

Everyone has a favorite meal or dessert, and any rigid diet eventually becomes too difficult to follow for a lifetime. I want you to change the majority of your choices and still have room for the occasional treat. Yes, you can have a little bit of wine. Once a week is OK, but don't drink the whole bottle. Don't drink wine every day, either. Give your body time to recover and filter out the toxins from the alcohol.

Once a month—say, on the first day or first weekend—enjoy the pleasure of the not-so-healthy foods you love. My patients in Brazil call it *festinha*, or "a little party." It's your limited time-out from the healthy diet, in which you step away from the rules without feeling guilty. You've been eating healthy all month, so you don't need to worry about one piece of cake or a favorite soda. Regularly eating a healthy diet allows you to splurge once in a while without significant consequences. But it's not a cheat day because you're not cheating. It's part of the plan, so there's no guilt involved!

Step 1: Make Sure You're Ready

If you're ill or have serious health conditions, first discuss the diet with your doctor. Also consider your timing. Don't make it more difficult on yourself by starting the day before a holiday feast, for instance. Before you start, ask yourself these questions:

- Am I in a good mental space to try something new?
- Do I have the support I need to start this reset?
- Am I OK with minor inconveniences?
- Do I have any major social events in the next 3 weeks?

- Do I have major travel plans in the next 3 weeks?
- Do I have the energy to create lists, answer questions, and reorganize my life right now?

Many people who follow the protocol report having more energy and clarity than before. If you start the diet and start to feel better, it might mean that something you were consuming was affecting your health. Before you start, take notes in your health journal about how you're sleeping and feeling overall. Having a starting reference point will help you appreciate the good you'll have done for your body.

If you slip, that's OK. Start over again. But sticking to the protocol consistently will make it faster and easier to reach your goals.

Step 2: Immunity Solution Diet Basics

Examine your labels and food sources. Avoid meals that aren't permitted or items that contain substances to avoid. Pay attention to your water, too. What you drink now will go into your cells today. The Immunity Solution Diet is alcohol-free, dairy-free, egg-free, fish-free, gluten-free, lab-free, nightshade-free, and pesticide-free. It requires self-control, so try to pack your food or eat at home during this short period. After 3 weeks, see how you feel. Self-imposed abstinence might even give you some new insights.

Foods to Eat

Animal fats such as duck fat, goose fat, lard, and tallow

Beef/steak (100 percent grass-fed)

Bone broth

Butter

Chicken (local, hormone-free, antibiotic-free, never-frozen)

Coconut oil

Fruits (low-sugar, local, non-GMO, pesticide-free), such as avocados,

blackberries, blueberries,
    lemons, limes
Kefir
Kimchi
Miso
Natto
Olive oil
Olives
Pickles

Sauerkraut
Vegetables (non-starch,
    local, non-GMO,
    pesticide-free), such
    as arugula, broccoli,
    cucumbers, and spinach
White rice (local, non-
    GMO, pesticide-free)
Yogurt (natural)

Beverages to Drink

Espresso (1 per
    day maximum)
Herbal tea

Mineral water (bottled
    in glass, not plastic)

Foods to Avoid

Crops not tested for
    biocides (pesticides,
    herbicides, etc.)
Eggs, lab-made eggs
Fake meats (lab-made)
Fish
Fruits from unknown
    sources

Genetically modified
    organisms (GMOs)
Lectins
Seed oils
Ultraprocessed food
Vegetable oils
Vegetables from
    unknown sources

Beverages to Avoid

Alcohol
Carbonated drinks
Coffee (unless organic)
Milk

Soda
Water from unknown
    sources (city,
    restaurant tap)

If you are prone to allergies, have an autoimmune condition, or immunity problems, stay away from spices, including ground peppercorns. Use Himalayan salt instead.

Because you're consuming much less sugar than before, you might feel hungrier in the first few days. That's normal, and eating more meat more often will combat that side effect. (Your energy levels might increase as another side effect.) The supplement section (page 223) discusses your nutrient needs and how to fulfill them in your diet.

SAMPLE MEAL PLANS

You can add any of the Foods to Eat or Beverages to Drink (pages 197–198) to these meals as long as they follow the stated rules.

Meal Plan 1

Breakfast: water, one espresso
Lunch: seared tri-tip steak
Dinner: grilled chicken wings
Snack: blueberries

Meal Plan 2

Breakfast: water, one espresso
Lunch: air-fried chicken breasts
Dinner: oven-roasted brisket
Snack: diced avocado drizzled with olive oil

Meal Plan 3

Breakfast: water, one espresso
Lunch: seared strip steak
Dinner: roasted lamb chops
Snack: lemon squares (recipe at ImmunitySolutionDiet.com)

Meal Plan 4

Breakfast: water, one espresso
Lunch: seared pork chops
Dinner: turkey burger patties
Snacks: bacon strips

Meal Plan 5

Breakfast: water, one espresso
Lunch: pan-fried beef meatballs with diced bacon
Dinner: seared filet mignon
Snack: homemade beef jerky

DAY 4: CHOOSE THE RIGHT MEAT

Most people enjoy eating meat, and the Immunity Solution Diet doesn't make you measure it because your body naturally will regulate your appetite as you embrace the protocol. Still, before beginning any new diet, check with your healthcare provider, especially if you have serious health conditions.

The most important point to know about eating meat is to check the sources. It sounds simple, but it isn't—especially with chicken. Before eating any piece of chicken, confirm that it's hormone-free. Chickens are naturally small birds. If a cut looks huge, chances are the bird didn't grow naturally.

DAY 5: FEED YOUR CELLS

Chances are that, as a child, you didn't learn how to feel healthy, happy, and energized through what you consumed. That's why it's difficult for you to know what to eat, how to eat, and why you eat at all. Your relationship with food probably reflects your attitudes toward yourself and those around you. Many people never learned to see food as a fuel source. Everything you eat and drink sooner or later feeds your cells, triggers your emotions, and shapes your health.

Every second of every day, our cells receive and transmit information. They respond to external stimuli very swiftly. Take, for example, the shock or fear triggered by the sight of a car crash or the delight at beholding puppies or kittens. Giving your cells the nutrients that they need drives the science of nutrition. Inside your body, each nutrient that you consume has a specific function, and your systems use or discard them based on what your body needs. Your various systems consist of various organs, which consist of various tissues, which consist of various cells. Those cells sustain your homeostasis. They support your body and mount an aggressive response against any potential threats. An army marches on its stomach, the old saying goes, so think of it like feeding an army. The better the food, the better the outcome. If you eat junk, you're going to feel like junk. If you eat well, you're going to feel well.

DAY 6: FEED YOUR JOY

This should go without saying, but it also bears repeating. When you feel good, keep doing what you're doing. Continue feeding your joy by making healthier, better choices for your overall health. Keep avoiding chemicals, pesticides, lab-created foods, ultraprocessed foods, and dangerous contaminants. Track what you're eating and how you're feeling. Be aware of any changes.

Bring your health journal to your next doctor's appointment so you can share your experience with your healthcare provider. We frequently rely on our memories, but memories betray us and rapidly fade. If you feel great—after a good night's sleep or an invigorating workout, for example—make a note that will inspire you going forward.

DAY 7: TRACK AND THINK

Before eating anything, know what you're eating and why. The point of this week is food awareness. Awareness of what and why you eat certain foods or drink specific beverages can help you see patterns. Are you reaching for chips at the end of a stressful day? Craving chocolate after talking to your boss or a client? Your mind and body are sending those cravings as messages about what's happening in your life. If you need to reduce the stress in your life, do that *before* inhaling the pint of ice cream.

Week 4.

SLEEP BETTER

SLEEP MIGHT NOT FEEL LIKE A SERIOUS ACTION STEP, BUT A LOT OF CRITICAL activity takes place in your body when you rest, including the production of molecules that fight infections. Getting enough sleep ensures good immune function. Sleep is just as important as food and water in your daily life for mental and physical functioning. In this step, you're going to follow the same routine and practice for the next 7 days.

BETTER SLEEP HABITS

Good sleep doesn't just happen the moment you decide that it's bedtime. Everything you do during the day leads to it. The following daily habits will lead to better rest at night.

Get Some Sun

Daylight has a strong influence on circadian rhythms. Daily exposure to sunlight will help synchronize your internal clock.

Burn Your Energy

Exercise benefits cardiovascular health and sleep quality. And you don't need to be a triathlete to reap the benefits. Even a moderate walk can help, and it's also a great way to get some daylight exposure. If you exercise heavily late in the day, finish at least an hour before going to bed to give your body time to wind down.

Nap

This one's not for everyone because not everyone likes napping. (I'm not a napper at all.) Some people can't sleep during the day or can't sleep anywhere other than their own beds. Napping too long can leave you feeling groggy and disoriented when you wake and interfere with your ability to sleep at night. Aim for short naps of no more than 20 to 30 minutes, no later than 3 p.m. Follow an abbreviated version of the sleep routine below. Give yourself time to wake up after a nap before returning to activities that require quick or sharp responses.

Limit Artificial Lights

Turn off the TV an hour before you want to be asleep. Dim indoor lighting with a dimmer or a low-watt lamp.

Reduce Screen Time

Smartphones and other devices can cause excessive mental stimulation or anxiety. They also emit blue light, which disrupts circadian rhythms. Avoid using all devices for at least an hour before bedtime.

Avoid Psychoactive Drugs

Caffeine, alcohol, and a wide range of medications contain psychoactive substances. For a good night's sleep, avoid alcohol and caffeine. Talk to your doctor about any medications that might be interfering with your rest.

Relax

It sounds simple, but in our go-go-go world, we often forget to relax. Techniques, such as a warm bath or yoga, can help you unwind, as can meditation and deep breathing. Before going to bed, avoid intense reading material. You want to unplug rather than activate your intellect.

DAYS 1 TO 7: READJUST YOUR SLEEP ROUTINE

Sleep schedules slip for everyone from time to time. Whether due to an urgent deadline, major travel, or caring for a newborn, temporary sleep disruption won't have long-term effects. But living long-term in a chronic sleep deficit will. To avoid a deficit, you must practice good sleep hygiene. Sometimes that requires retraining your body to sleep. Here are a few steps for better sleep or a new bedtime routine.

Step 1: Create a New Routine

Before you begin your routine, set your alarm, not to wake up but to go to bed. First, determine how many hours of sleep you typically need to feel rested. Then work backward from your morning routines and commitments to give yourself the necessary time, which will help you avoid sleep inertia as well. It may seem strange at first, but your body will adjust to this new habit in no time, and good sleep will become your new normal. At 9:30 p.m., my phone reminds me of my bedtime, and that's when I head to bed, put on a sleep mask, and go to sleep. Most days, I wake at 4:30 a.m., no alarm, when my body feels ready. Try it yourself. You will love feeling refreshed with no alarms and no surprises.

Most parents create a bedtime routine for young children: bath, book or story, lights out. The sequence teaches them to wind down and rest. Adults need the same practice. Consistent cues can have a big psychological impact on routines. To prepare for your new routine, invest in an eye mask (black or dark-colored for maximum light blocking); herbal teas, such as chamomile, valerian, or other sleepy teas; small doses of a trusted melatonin supplement; and a white noise machine, playlist, or app.

Routine

- Set a nightly alarm to go to bed.
- If you can, set your bedroom temperature to around 68°F.
- Take a warm bath (or shower if you don't have a tub).
- Make a cup of caffeine-free herbal tea.
- Put on the white noise machine, playlist, or app for 15 minutes while drinking the tea.
- Brush your teeth.
- Stretch and put on pajamas.
- Dim the lights in your sleeping space and read quietly for 15 to 30 minutes.
- Put on your eye mask and lie down.
- Mentally thank someone who made you happy today. Let your mind wander.
- Relax. Enjoy the comfort of your bed.

Week 5.

MOVE YOUR BODY

KEEPING FIT IS ESSENTIAL FOR GOOD HEALTH, BUT HOW SHOULD YOU DO THAT effectively? Exercise alone rarely will help you lose weight because the more calories you burn, the more fuel your body craves to reach its natural equilibrium. You can't outrun, outlift, or out-swim a bad diet or other negative habits, so don't use exercise as a substitute for making healthy choices.

Physical fitness does improve your circulation, however, which allows all your cells, including your army of immune cells, to move faster and more freely throughout your body to scan for trouble. Regular moderate exercise reduces inflammation and helps immune cells regenerate. In people with weakened defenses, even one sensible exercise session can increase vaccine effectiveness.

As you age, you should be strengthening your core, legs, and arms and working on your balance. If you're short on time or can't make it to the gym, try these seven simple exercises. Begin with 3 sets of 10 reps of each exercise. As you build strength, create a full-body circuit workout by mixing and matching them as you like. Remember that people who exercise in the morning have a better chance at staying consistent than people who exercise at the end of the day. Whether you join a gym or follow a class online or on TV, the important part is to keep moving for your physical health and well-being.

DAY 1: LUNGES

This exercise strengthens your legs and butt muscles. It also builds your balance, key for aging independently.

1.   Stand with your feet hip-width apart.
2.   Place your right leg slightly ahead of your body and your left slightly behind it.
3.   Keeping your left foot in place, step forward with your right leg, longer than a walking stride.
4.   Your right foot should land flat on the ground. Your left heel will rise off the ground.
5.   Lower your body, bending your knees to about 90 degrees. Don't let your right knee go past your right foot.
6.   Keep your core engaged and your torso upright.
7.   Rise, returning to the starting position.
8.   Repeat with the opposite leg.

DAY 2: PUSH-UPS

This exercise works every muscle in your body. If you have trouble doing standard push-ups, start with modified push-ups, knees on the ground.

1.   Position yourself on all fours on the floor. Place your hands slightly wider than your shoulders.
2.   Keep your elbows slightly bent, not locked and straight.

3. Extend your legs back until your hands and toes balance your weight. Position your feet hip-width apart.

4. Tighten your core by pulling your belly button inward toward your spine.

5. Inhale as you lower yourself to the floor, slowly bending your elbows until they form a 90-degree angle.

6. Exhale as you push up through your hands, feeling your chest muscles contract and returning to the starting position.

7. Repeat.

DAY 3: STAR CROSS TOUCHES

You can do this easy, whole-body stretch anytime. It works your shoulders, core, butt, and legs all at the same time.

1. Stand with your feet shoulder-width apart.

2. Raise your arms to the sides, forming a star with your whole body.

3. Keeping your legs as straight as possible, bend forward from the hips so your back is parallel to the ground.

4. Bring your right arm down and across to your left foot while reaching upward with your left arm. Look up at your left hand as you twist.

5. In reverse order—arms then back—return to the starting position.

6. Repeat on the other side.

DAY 4: REST

If you exercise regularly, you need one rest day per week to heal tissues, develop muscle, and replenish fuel reserves. Rest days also help alleviate emotional stress. Instead of a work-out today, go for an easy walk, followed by a warm bath with Epsom salts, which help replace magnesium stores and reduce muscle swelling.

DAY 5: JUMPING SQUATS

This exercise strengthens your core and lower body and makes your hips and legs more flexible. It also burns a lot of calories because it works your largest muscles.

1. Stand with your feet hip-width apart, toes slightly pointed out.
2. Clasp your hands at your chest for balance.
3. Bend your knees, lowering yourself as far as possible. Don't bend your knees more than 90 degrees or let your knees extend past your toes. Keep your chest vertical. Tighten your butt to keep your hips from pitching forward.
4. Release your hands and swing your arms down to generate momentum.
5. Press through your heels and jump as fast as you can.
6. Gently touch down and return to a squat position.
7. Repeat.

DAY 6: SIT-UPS

Full sit-ups strengthen your abdominal muscles easily and effectively. If you have lower back pain or you can't lift your back all the way off the ground, do crunches instead, which call for lifting only your shoulders and upper back. Putting your hands behind your head can strain your neck and deisolate your abs, so don't do that.

1. Lie on the floor on your back.

2. Bend your knees and place your feet flat on the ground.

3. If necessary, tuck your feet under a bench, piece of furniture, or other support.

4. Cross your arms over your chest, left hand on right shoulder and vice versa.

5. Activate your core by pulling your belly button inward toward your spine.

6. Slowly lift your back off the ground using only your abdominal muscles. Keep your tailbone and hips still and pressed into the floor.

7. Lower yourself slowly back to the starting position. Don't let your head or back thud on the floor.

8. Repeat.

DAY 7: YOGA

Great for stretching your body and controlling your breath, yoga offers a wide variety of approaches and practices aimed at uniting body, mind, and spirit. In the West, just "yoga" usually means hatha yoga, one of the numerous types. Hatha yoga uses *asanas* (poses), *pranayama* (breathing), *mudra* (gestures), and *shatkarma* (self-discipline) to create an inside-outside unity. It cleanses the body and cultivates *prana* (life force energy). Most yoga practices don't emphasize the more esoteric sides of hatha yoga, concentrating instead on the poses, which offer fantastic training for strength and balance. The more you practice it, though, the more it will benefit your abilities to breathe, meditate, and relax.

Yoga usually takes place barefoot on a sticky yoga mat with optional supports. The poses and moves require clothing that can stretch and move freely with your body. You can buy yoga-specific attire, but you probably can assemble an appropriate outfit from your existing wardrobe. Some yoga courses use props, such as straps, blocks, blankets, or bolsters, but you can improvise at home with scarves, neckties, stacks of books, or cushions. Most studios have extra props for class use.

Try yoga today. Find a studio, a practice in your neighborhood, or even a video online. (Sites such as Yoga with Adrienne have free videos for all levels with thorough instructions.) All you need is comfortable clothes, a mat (if the studio doesn't provide one), and some water for after your workout. Begin with a short, simple class and work your way up from there. Once you've mastered the fundamental beginner poses, you can put them together into a sequence and progress to more difficult poses.

If you don't like yoga or the idea of it, follow a comprehensive stretching program or another low-impact, full-body exercise that you enjoy.

Week 6.

CALM YOUR MIND

WELCOME TO ZEN WEEK! MOST PEOPLE SPEND SO MUCH OF THEIR LIVES building their résumés or sprinting toward life goals that they forget what really matters: time. It's the most valuable asset you have. If you often lose track of it and become hyperfocused on details that truly don't matter, it's time to unwind, relax, and rekindle. Every day this week, you'll focus on strategies to help reorganize skewed priorities, ways to reduce stress, and practices to help you find calm in any storm. Try each of them and see which ones work best for you. Do whatever works to calm your mind and help you find your center again. If you have to do it a few times throughout a stressful day, that's OK. Once you've determined your favorites, put them into daily practice for 21 days to solidify that new, positive habit.

DAY 1: REFRAME YOUR PERSPECTIVE

As a cancer doctor, I have witnessed death up close many times. Patients on their deathbeds look at life with a different perspective. People whose lives are hanging in the balance can't think in terms of years. They can keep tabs on weeks, however. Whether you have 200 or 2,000 before you reach the end of the road, it works just the same. With that in mind, my advice for you is to measure your life in weeks, not years. That new framework will prompt you to make changes now, as necessary, rather than some undetermined point in the future. If you want to spend time with loved ones, pursue a passion, or find true love, set those goals in terms of weeks.

Step 1: Memento Mori

Translated from Latin, *memento mori* means "remembrance of death." As a meditative exercise, it can help you find your center and determine your priorities. When all is quiet and still in your home, take a moment to think about your death. How do you imagine it? How will people remember you? What legacy do you want to leave? The more vividly you can imagine specific details, the better the exercise works. It may seem morbid, but pondering life's end can help you identify your real priorities. Maybe in picturing your death you see your children, sad that you didn't spend more time with them while they were growing up or that they didn't get to know you as well as you would have liked. If so, perhaps you're spending too much time working and not enough time with them.

You can regret or dwell on mistakes, but the past is gone. Put it out of mind. Maybe you failed at something—that's OK. Life is short, and we can't control so much of it. Sorrow ages people quickly. Focus on what lies next in your path. Practicing memento mori will keep you grounded and humble, reminding you how brief life is and how important it is to follow what matters. It also will help you recontextualize everyday annoyances or problems. Whatever inconvenience or challenge you're facing will end one day, too, just like all the other weeks you have pushed through and survived. All storms pass, and the sun will shine again.

DAY 2: SEPARATE YOURSELF FROM YOUR JOB OR CAREER

It's hard to find people who don't consider themselves very busy. Whether you're running the kids to recitals or practice, trying to make partner at a major law firm, or both, our increasingly frenetic world probably is pushing you to focus on mundane preoccupations, like social status or chasing the latest trends. Even retirees complain of having too much to do.

To date, I have delivered 23 babies into this world, and I have held the hands of far too many people on their deathbeds. The people who were dying shared three main regrets. None of them wished they'd done more video meetings or had better year-end reviews. To a person, they wished that they had done more of what made them happy, spent more time with loved ones, and taken the risk to chase their dreams.

It's so easy to fall into the stress of the here and now. A work crisis hits, the WiFi goes down, the plane gets delayed, all leaving you feeling mad and producing more cortisol than your body needs. When you finally take a break, ready to enjoy some peace and quiet, you catch a cold or the flu. Maybe a pipe bursts and floods your kitchen. What do you do? Do you lose it or take a moment to laugh at the random absurdity of reality? One day, your employer could close up shop, or your job could become automated. Those possibilities will affect your livelihood, sure, but stressing over them does more harm than good. Someone did your job or one just like it before you, and someone will do it or one just like it after you. Everyone is replaceable. In the meantime, every stomach-churningly stressful minute is damaging your immune system.

Identifying closely with your career isn't bad in and of itself, but it can make you vulnerable in a variety of ways. Burning out, getting laid off, or even retiring can send your mind into an unhealthy loop. If you lose perspective of what matters most to you, you can develop needless anxiety or depression. By reasserting yourself as a person first and a smart or hard worker second, you can build a more balanced, healthy life.

Step 1: Delegate

All tasks fall into three categories of importance: high, medium, and low. All tasks also fall into three time frames for completion: quick, average, and time-consuming. While you're focusing on urgent matters that you can knock out quickly, delegate low-importance tasks that are time-consuming. You might need to enlist the help of junior colleagues, hire a virtual assistant, or request an intern. Effective delegation necessitates relinquishing some control over how the work will be completed, which is a healthy exercise in communication and acceptance in and of itself.

Step 2: Reframe Your Skills

Rethink your relationship with your job. If you had to leave your industry tomorrow, what would you do? What new jobs or careers could you pursue right away? Think of what you do not as an identity or title but in terms of skills applicable in a variety of situations. Many psychotherapists, for example, have skills that translate well to human resources or guidance counseling.

DAY 3: KNOW WHAT'S IMPORTANT

I grew up in Brazil and worked on the outskirts of São Paulo. Visiting patients in the favelas there exposed me to realities difficult to comprehend even now. The same society that had afforded me the opportunity to study medicine and buy new shoes whenever I needed or wanted left many people without access to clean water or basic nourishment.

One patient call brought me to a tiny home made of clay, about an hour away from São Paulo's city center. In the small space, the pungent scent of bacterial infection filled my nostrils. Someone inside was very sick. In a chair sat a man certainly older than 80, but he couldn't tell me for sure because he himself didn't know his own birthdate. He had a foot infection that was spreading quickly, and he needed hospital-grade antibiotics. We immediately transported him to the nearest hospital. During the ride, I was administering IV fluids to him when he told me that he was the son of slaves.

Slaves? It seemed impossible. The old man said that his mother had been kept hostage for her entire life on a farm not far from where he lived. He had escaped many years ago, but she died in captivity. Brazil abolished slavery in 1888, but in some places the despicable practice continued in secret. I had no idea that people still were being enslaved in my own country. His shocking revelation broke my heart and gave me perspective that I've never forgotten.

He wasn't resentful or angry. He was content with his life, grateful for the medical help, and happy to see another sunrise. He didn't focus on his poverty or his past. He was living in a moment of gratitude. Some people call it emotional intelligence, having perspective, or seeing the big picture. The phrase itself doesn't matter. It's about not becoming too attached to what you can't control and understanding the preciousness of every moment you have.

Step 1: Decide What Matters

Reflect on your belief systems, principles, and values. What matters most to you? Make a list of what you couldn't live without. You can start with the basics—water, food, money—then identify the most important people and passions in your life. By clarifying your values, you determine what to embrace further and what you can let go. Let your priorities lead you to the next step. Consider your goals in areas such as parenting, relationships, community, and career. Rank them in order of importance. Formal worksheets can help organize your thoughts, but you also can keep a running list on your phone or in your health journal as you ponder your most important priorities.

DAY 4: CALM YOUR MIND

It takes time to develop different ways to manage stress, so don't give up too quickly. Shifting focus from stressors to intentional rhythms requires dedication, but it can strengthen your mental and emotional stamina. If you need more help getting a handle on your stress, don't be afraid to seek professional help.

Step 1: Take It Easy

If you find yourself checking work email on nights or weekends, stop. Try some new hobbies unrelated to work or anything else you're doing already, such as baking, calligraphy, gardening, knitting, painting, or photography. If you want to learn a new language but Spanish feels like work because your company deals with a lot of clients in Latin America, pursue French instead. You don't have to make a long-term commitment, either. The point is to do something new and have fun. If you want to get more exercise, don't sign up for a marathon. Try hitting the gym at lunchtime for some light strength training or, if you can, walk or bike home from work a couple of times a week. It's easier to implement and maintain small changes, which, over time, can lead to a virtuous cycle of commitment and self-improvement.

Step 2: Connect with Others

During the pandemic, we all spent so many hours alone, craving social connection for our own mental health. Reenergize your social circles by attending community events, joining local clubs or organizations, and making some new friends. You'll have a good time while forming a new support system. Reaching out to people with whom you've lost touch also can help reconnect you to a healthier version of yourself. It doesn't take much. Recent research on adult friendships indicates that having just three to five close friends correlates with the highest levels of life satisfaction.

DAY 5: MEDITATE

Meditation has consisted of a variety of practices and techniques for thousands of years. Regardless of which you pursue, you need to understand how and why it works in easing your mental space. Most practices encourage you to fix your mind on a chosen objective when meditating, which is why some people employ mantras. Other people, including me, prefer candle gazing.

Reaching a meditative state doesn't require you to embrace collective consciousness or lose your sense of self. It's not about controlling or mastering your mind. Meditation can help you achieve a deep state of neutral relaxation. It starts with unplugging from notifications and requests and being fully present. It turns off what some psychologists call the "monkey mind," that constant troop of anxiety and worries that creates mental chaos. When you meditate, you sweep that disorder away. The goal is to become unseen, unreachable, silent—even if only for 10 minutes.

You already have the tools to meditate and use them, too. Your reticular activating system (RAS) determines how you perceive and react to the external world. It regulates your wakefulness, ability to focus, and fight-flight-or-freeze response. In broad terms, it controls your consciousness, gatekeeping all the data you collect through your various senses. In a loud restaurant, with a good friend or significant other, you can tune out all the extraneous noise to concentrate on your conversation, right? That's your RAS in action. It allows your mind to work in the background, keeping your systems active without bombarding them with constant sensory input. Your RAS creates an intentional filter for your focus of choice. It sorts through the sensory input and displays only what's relevant. You can harness the power of your RAS to focus on the moment and ignore everything else.

Step 1: Candle Meditation

This technique is great for beginners. Get any kind of candle and light it. Dim the lights so the flame becomes the focal point of the room. Place the candle on a table and sit in front of it. For ease and comfort, try to place the flame at eye level, approximately 2 feet away. Keep your back straight to allow your diaphragm a full range of motion. Set a timer for 10 or 15 minutes. Take a couple of deep, slow breaths. Relax and release any tension in your body. Focus solely on the flame. Observe as it flickers, changes shape, emits a halo, and flashes a variety of colors. If your mind wanders, don't worry. Just lead it back to the flame. You may have to corral your mind several times. The more you practice it, the easier it becomes.

DAY 6: BREATHE

When you breathe in, blood cells receive oxygen and release carbon dioxide, the waste product you exhale. Abdominal breathing, belly breathing, diaphragmatic breathing, and paced respiration all describe deep breathing. When you take a deep breath, air completely fills your lungs and your lower belly rises. When you don't breathe deeply, you limit your diaphragm's range of motion, and the bottom part of your lungs doesn't receive enough oxygenated air. You may feel out of breath or anxious as a result. Breathing problems can cause fatigue, panic attacks, and other physical and emotional problems because they disrupt the exchange of oxygen and carbon dioxide. Deep breathing, on the other hand, can lower or stabilize your blood pressure while also slowing your heartbeat.

To do this exercise, all you really need to do is breathe deeply and slowly with intention. Once you've mastered that simple practice, here are three more ways to breathe for calmness.

Step 1: Alternate-Nostril Breathing

Sit upright and maintain your posture. Close your eyes or gaze downward. Inhale and exhale once, as normal, then close your right nostril with your thumb. Inhale through your left nostril and hold the breath. Close your left nostril and open your right nostril. Exhale through the right nostril. Inhale through your right nostril and hold the breath. Close your right nostril with your thumb, release your left nostril, and exhale through your left nostril.

Complete 10 rounds of this breathing pattern. Take a break if you feel dizzy. Breathe normally after releasing both nostrils.

Step 2: 4-7-8 Breathing

This exercise naturally relaxes your nervous system. Until you master it, do it seated with your back straight. After that, you can do it while lying in bed.

Place the tip of your tongue against the ridge of tissue behind your upper front teeth. Completely exhale through your mouth, making a *whoosh* sound. Close your mouth and inhale quietly through your nose to a mental count of four. Hold your breath for a count of seven. Exhale completely through your mouth, making a *whoosh* sound again, to a count of eight. Repeat three times.

Step 3: Lion's Breath

This deep breathing technique, called *simhasana* in Sanskrit, can help relax your face and jaw muscles, relieve stress, and improve your cardiovascular function. Sit, leaning forward slightly, with your hands on your knees or the floor. Spread your fingers as wide as possible across your knees. Inhale through your nose. Open your mouth wide, stick out your tongue, and point it down toward your chin. Exhale forcefully, carrying the breath across the root of your tongue. While exhaling, make a "ha" sound from deep within your abdomen. Breathe normally for a few moments. Repeat Lion's Breath up to seven times.

DAY 7: ACHIEVE RELEASE

At the end of your Zen week, calm your mind with another simple yet effective practice. In a quiet place in your home or office, gather two small pieces of paper. On the first one, write down something that recently caused you distress. It can be the weather, traffic, your boss, a client—anything that caused you frustration. Set the paper aside. On the second piece of paper, write down something that brought you joy, such as a smile from a stranger, good news in an email, the food you ate, or anything that made your heart sing.

Place both pieces of paper side by side and say, "Thank you" aloud. Acknowledge that both events happened, the good and the not so good. Dispose of both papers however you prefer, taking a second to release the energy of whatever happened that day.

Week 7.

SUPPLEMENT BETTER

BY NOW, YOUR BODY'S READY FOR SOME GOOD VITAMINS AND ADAPTOGENS to kick-start the last week of the Immunity Solution Protocol and the next phase of your life. If you think that megadosing certain vitamins will improve your immune system, think again. Too much of anything can cause harm. Vitamin B complex, C, D, multivitamins, mushroom supplements, and zinc in the proper amounts all promote immune system function. Other supplements help, too.

DAYS 1 TO 7: DETERMINE YOUR DEFICIENCIES

If you're not tracking the nutritional content of your diet already, you should be. Remember, information is power. This is another point where your health journal can come in handy.

Step 1: Do the Math

Track what you eat every day this week. Look at the macronutrients (carbs, fat, protein) as well as micronutrients (vitamins and minerals). See how you compare with the FDA recommended daily intake for each category. If you're not getting enough of something, consider adjusting your diet or taking an appropriate supplement.

Step 2: Look at Your Levels

All bodies differ, and some absorb nutrients differently than others. Many doctors now post bloodwork results to an online patient portal. If yours does, go look at the numbers there and see how your levels compare to healthy ranges. Again, consider adjusting your diet or taking the corresponding supplement.

Step 3: Supplement Questionnaire

Before you go on a supplement shopping spree, answer the following questions.

- Have you ever used supplements before? Why?
- How many pills are you comfortable taking every day?
- Have you ever tried powders in the past?
- Are you willing to try CBD tinctures or oils to reduce stress?
- Do you add proteins, collagens, or other powders to your beverages?
- Are you trying to stay away from vegetable and seed oils?
- Are you trying to avoid soy, wheat, and other crops?
- Do you find yourself running low on energy at the end of the day?
- Do you have any known allergies?

Taking the right supplements can help, but they aren't all good. Eating natural, organic food provides the best source of all nutrients. If you don't have the perfect diet, though, supplementation may be right for you. Seek immune-friendly formulations and also check with your doctor because prescription supplements have been vetted rigorously for quality, unlike their OTC counterparts.

Maintenance:

CELLULAR FEEDING

CONGRATULATIONS! YOU'VE FINISHED THE 7-WEEK IMMUNITY SOLUTION PRO-tocol. Now it's time to enter the maintenance phase, your life-long commitment to healthier choices, a stronger immune system, and better health. You've developed positive new habits for stress, exercise, and sleep, so continue those great practices for a lifetime of balanced mental and physical wellness.

For the nutritional component, the restrictive aspects of the Immunity Solution Diet might make it difficult to maintain long-term, but you also don't want to lose the gains you've made. That's where cellular feeding comes into play. This science-based method of deliberate eating alters your psychological connection to what you eat, when, and why. It blends research, traditional practices, and meditation to shift your mindset about food. But it's not a diet. Most diets fail because people hate to diet. Even the word some-times creates resistance.

Cellular feeding invites you to understand how your body

works, how to be healthy without dieting, and how to live better by feeding your cells and your soul. Everything you consume fuels your cells. The water you drink, the food you eat, and the supplements you take constantly impact your internal interactions at a molecular level. As you know after eating a greasy or spicy meal, your body reacts differently to different types of nutrition. It wants from you, at the most basic level, the power to work effectively. Cellular feeding doesn't restrict what you can consume but rather points you toward foods and beverages that make you feel better, happier, and healthier.

Step 1: Eat with Intention and Purpose

Before consuming anything, think carefully about what it is and why you want it. Ask yourself: What will this do for my body? It's OK to eat for pleasure once in a while. Those indulgences make life worth living. But now that you've created a healthier relationship with yourself, you don't want to sabotage it accidently. Your two main concerns should be: Does this feed my cells? Does this feed my soul?

If you're not sure, think about it in terms of long-term survival, maintenance, health, and healing. Will this help you live longer? Will this help you maintain your health? Will this help you heal? In that context, these two, simple yes-or-no questions can help you regain self-control while also living your life to the fullest. They allow you to reset your health at any moment without worrying about calories or how much you weigh.

Revisit the allowed Immunity Solution Diet foods (page 195) anytime you like. If you need a little more help, as we all sometimes do, follow these general guidelines.

CATEGORY	AVOID	CONSUME
Animal Protein	Chicken from unknown sources, mercury-rich fish such as salmon and tuna	Grass-fed beef, humanely raised pork, chicken free of antibiotics and hormones
Vegetable Protein	Whey protein, peanuts, and soy	Organic, non-GMO beans and other legumes
Grains and Starches	Corn and wheat	Organic, non-GMO rice and sweet potatoes
Vegetables	Anything frozen or store-bought, nightshades (eggplant, potatoes, tomatoes), and peas	Organic, non-GMO beets, carrots, and asparagus
Fruits	Anything frozen or store-bought, oranges, strawberries	Organic, non-GMO apples, apricots, blueberries, cranberries, peaches, pears, and pineapples
Sweeteners	Sugar, maple syrup, fructose	Sucralose and stevia
Dairy	2-percent, low-fat, or fat-free milk, or ultraprocessed milk by-products	Butter, whole milk, and whole-milk products
Beverages	City water, water from unknown sources, carbonation, alcohol	Organic, non-GMO coffee and teas, mineral water

You already have a decent notion of what you can eat and what you should avoid. It isn't nearly as complicated as it might feel. For better health, self-control is key. Give yourself some wiggle room with the occasional treat for your soul, but don't make a habit of it.

Try not to snack, which usually is satisfying cravings in the brain, not the stomach. Dieting for weight loss can prove effective in some situations, but it's easier to achieve the same results when you tailor your intake to the needs of your body, rather than your mind.

NOT AT HOME

Patients often ask what to do when going out to eat, attending a party, or participating in an event that gives them no control over the nourishment available. The strategy is simple. Those situations are outliers. They shouldn't occur frequently nor become habits. In those cases, feed your soul in healthy moderation. Remember, life is about balance, not rigidity.

Step 2: Follow the Protocol

Hopefully the 7-week protocol gave you a fresh perspective. To maintain the health you've restored to your body, regularly reevaluate your daily rituals, practices, and behaviors. You know better now and have experienced how good it feels to live healthily. Keep reading the labels on anything that comes into contact with your body, including personal care products. Remember, your skin is your largest organ, it's highly permeable, and it contains lots of immune cells. What it touches matters.

After committing to just 3 weeks of going nicotine-free, many people decide to quit. When I was younger, smoking became a habit during the rigors of medical school. When I pursued a career in cancer research, I saw the foolishness of continuing to smoke. For 3 weeks, I didn't have a single cigarette. After those 21 days, it felt mentally easier to quit than if I had committed to quitting cold turkey forever. That mind hack gave me the help I needed.

If you struggled to abstain from alcohol, consider reevaluating your connection with it. Not everyone needs to avoid it completely, but you need to know who's in charge. When you lose your self-control, addictions take over. An occasional indulgence can become an addiction, so make sure that you're not using alcohol or any other substance as a crutch to get through life. As with anything, moderation is key.

As you reflect on your daily habits, try to continue taking notes—in additional health journals or elsewhere—because that step gives you a record of your life and makes taking meaningful action much easier. Too many people reach places of no return with their health and wish, too late, that they had done things differently. That doesn't have to be you. You now have the knowledge, tools, and guidance to change your future. The power lies in your hands. Make the most of every minute. Each one has the potential to be your most valuable moment.

ACKNOWLEDGMENTS

A book isn't just words; it's a collection of yeses from people who agree to embark on a journey with you. It all begins with your parents, your true first teachers, guiding you as you start to experience the world. It continues, if you're lucky, throughout your life with other masters, friends, and professors. In this life, it seems that the teacher always shows up right when the student is ready. Here, I thank a select group of people who agreed to work on my projects, encouraged me along the way, and made it possible for me to speak my thoughts into existence. Without you, none of this would have been possible, so please accept my heartfelt gratitude.

To the University of Texas MD Anderson Cancer Center, whose mission to #endcancer is achieved on a daily basis, as well as the Parker Institute for Cancer Immunotherapy, whose research has resulted in groundbreaking discoveries.

Special thanks to Padmanee Sharma and James P. Allison, whose work challenged the status quo of medical science, altered the course of history, and saved hundreds of thousands of lives. Standing in your shadows is a blessing.

To Brian Wallach, who is the most amazing human being alive, devoting his minutes, hours, and days to the benefit of others. If only we could have more Brian Wallachs in the world, we might be able to achieve true peace on earth.

To my loving family: my grandmother Maria Salvador Nissola, who endured so much and yet had so much joy to give; my grandmother Tereza Rosa Florindo, who always had a smile to give and words of wisdom to share; my uncle João Roberto Florindo, who taught me that life should be a game of love, laughter, and excitement; and always to my loving parents, Ana Rosa Nissola and Ivo Nissola, who wholeheartedly supported my educational endeavors and taught me unconditional love.

Many mentors inspired and encouraged me in my work and life. Sumit Subudhi, MD, PhD, is the best oncologist I know; Ramy Ibrahim, MD, is the best drug developer I know; Monica Mazzurana, MD, has the best bedside manner I have ever seen; Ricardo Cunegundes, MD, was a wonderful boss; and Bruno Pagnoncelli, MD, has taught me so much more than just medicine. John Tass-Parker once saved my life from a mountaintop blizzard.

Dozens of people have propelled me forward in life and with this project. It's impossible to list them all, but I'll give a shout out to a very special few: the incredible Ana Carolina Porto, MD, whom I miss every day; Bruna Mara Paiva, MD, who always takes my midnight calls; Beatriz Dalpino, the perfect example of discipline and kindness; Wendy Guarisco and Kelly George, whose work made it all possible; the wonderful Deb Swacker, whose energy lights up the world; Clare Gannon and Jano Cabrera, who have adopted me as their own; Scott Mulhauser, the best buddy I could ask for; Nate Rawlings, who graciously edited my first national opinion piece; Shirley Jump, who is a word magician; and Sandra Abrevaya, whose meticulous research skills should be taught in medical schools across the globe. Special thanks to Pamela Harty, my agent, and James Jayo, my editor at Countryman.

These people have shaped much of the framework of my life and my work. Without them, I wouldn't be who I am today. A simple thank-you isn't enough to repay your support.

NOTES

1. "Antibiotic Resistant Bacteria," Victoria State Government, Better Health Channel, https://www.betterhealth.vic.gov.au/health/conditionsandtreatments/antibiotic-resistant-bacteria.

2. Bruce Alberts, Alexander Johnson, Julian Lewis, et al, *Helper T-Cells and Lymphocyte Activation* (New York: Garland Science, 2002), https://www.ncbi.nlm.nih.gov/books/NBK26827.

3. David D. Chaplin, "Overview of the Immune Response, " *The Journal of Allergy and Clinical Immunology* 125, no. 2 Suppl 2 (February 2010): S3–23, https://doi.org/10.1016/j.jaci.2009.12.980.

4. Genetic Alliance and District of Columbia Department of Health, *Newborn Screening* (Washington, DC: Genetic Alliance, 2010), 19–30, https://www.ncbi.nlm.nih.gov/books/NBK132148.

5. Kurt Whittemore, Elsa Vera, Eva Martínez-Nevado, et al, "Telomere Shortening Rate Predicts Species Life Span," *Proceedings of the National Academy of Sciences of the United States of America* 116, no. 30 (July 23, 2019): 15122–27, https://doi.org/10.1073/pnas.1902452116.

6. Johns Hopkins Medicine, "Accurate telomere length test influences treatment decisions for certain diseases," ScienceDaily, www.sciencedaily.com/releases/2018/02/180226122522.htm.

7. Marjorie K. Jeffcoat, Robert L. Jeffcoat, Patricia A. Gladowski, et al, "Impact of Periodontal Therapy on General Health: Evidence from Insurance Data for Five Systemic Conditions," *American Journal of Preventive Medicine* 47, no. 2 (August 1, 2014): 166–74, https://doi.org/10.1016/j.amepre.2014.04.001.

8. "The Brain-Gut Connection," Hopkins Medicine, last modified November 1, 2021, https://www.hopkinsmedicine.org/health/wellness-and-prevention/the-brain-gut-connection.

9. Thomas C. Fung, Helen E. Vuong, Cristopher D. G. Luna, et al, "Intestinal Serotonin and Fluoxetine Exposure Modulate Bacterial Colonization in the Gut," *Nature Microbiology* 4, no. 12 (December 2019): 2064–73, https://doi.org/10.1038/s41564-019-0540-4.

10. Jessica M. Yano, Kristie Yu, Gregory P. Donaldson, et al, "Indigenous Bacteria from the Gut Microbiota Regulate Host Serotonin Biosynthesis," *Cell* 161, no. 2 (April 9, 2015): 264–76, https://doi.org/10.1016/j.cell.2015.02.047.

11. Mun-Keat Looi, "The Human Microbiome: Everything You Need to Know About the 39 Trillion Microbes That Call Our Bodies Home," *BBC Science Focus*, July 14, 2020, https://www.sciencefocus.com/the-human-body/human-microbiome/.

12. Amy D. Proal, Paul J. Albert, Trevor G. Marshall, "The Human Microbiome and Autoimmunity," *Current Opinion in Rheumatology* 25, no. 2 (March 2013): 234–40, https://doi.org/10.1097/BOR.0b013e32835cedbf.

13. Luba Vikhanski, "A Science Lecture Accidentally Sparked a Global Craze for Yogurt," *Smithsonian Magazine*, April 11 206, https://www.smithsonianmag.com/science-nature/science-lecture-accidentally-sparked-global-craze-yogurt-180958700/.

14. US Food & Drug Administration Office of Criminal Investigation, "GNC Enters Into Agreement with Department of Justice to Improve Its Practices and Keep Potentially Illegal Dietary Supplements Out of the Marketplace," US Department of Justice Press Release, December 7, 2016, https://www.fda.gov/inspections-compliance-enforcement-and-criminal-investigations/press-releases/december-7-2016-gnc-enters-agreement-department-justice-improve-its-practices-and-keep-potentially.

15. Snigdha Vallabhaneni, Tiffany A. Walker, Shawn R. Lockhart, et al, "Fatal Gastrointestinal Mucormycosis in a Premature Infant Associated with a Contaminated Dietary Supplement—Connecticut, 2014," *Morbidity and Mortality Weekly Report* 64, no. 6 (February 20, 2015): 155–56, https://www.ncbi.nlm.nih.gov/pmc/articles/PMC4584706/.

16. Isabelle Meyts, Aziz Bousfiha, Carla Duff, et al, "Primary Immunodeficiencies: A Decade of Progress and a Promising Future," *Frontiers in Immunology* 11 (2020): 625753, https://doi.org/10.3389/fimmu.2020.625753.

17. National Institutes of Health, "Autoimmunity May Be Rising in the United States," NIH News Release, April 8, 2020, https://www.nih.gov/news-events/news-releases/autoimmunity-may-be-rising-united-states.

18. James Dahlgren, Harpreet Takhar, Pamela Anderson-Mahoney, et al, "Cluster of Systemic Lupus Erythematosus (SLE) Associated with an Oil Field Waste Site: A Cross Sectional Study," *Environmental Health* 6, no. 8 (2007), https://doi.org/10.1186/1476-069X-6-8.

19. "Lupus Linked to Petroleum Exposure." Newsdesk.org, May 23, 2007, http://newsdesk.org/2007/05/23/lupus_linked_to/.

20. Aram Mokarizadeh, Mohammad Reza Faryabi, Mohammad Amin Rezvanfar, et al, "A Comprehensive Review of Pesticides and the Immune Dysregulation: Mechanisms, Evidence and Consequences," *Toxicology Mechanisms and Methods* 25, no. 4 (May 4, 2015): 258–78, https://doi.org/10.3109/15376516.2015.1020182.

21. "Diagnosing Autoimmune Diseases," Benaroya Research Institute, October 20, 2017, https://www.benaroyaresearch.org/blog/post/diagnosing-autoimmune-diseases.

22. Arndt Manzel, Dominik N. Muller, David A. Hafler, et al, "Role of 'Western Diet' in Inflammatory Autoimmune Diseases," *Current Allergy and Asthma Reports* 14, no. 1 (January 2014): 404, https://doi.org/10.1007/s11882-013-0404-6.

23. Yiliang Wang, Zhaoyang Wang, Yun Wang, et al, "The Gut-Microglia Connection: Implications for Central Nervous System Diseases," *Frontiers in Immunology* 9 (October 5, 2018): 2325, https://doi.org/10.3389/fimmu.2018.02325.

24. Luigi Naldi, "Psoriasis and Smoking: Links and Risks," *Psoriasis: Targets and Therapy* 6 (May 2016): 65–71, https://doi.org/10.2147/PTT.S85189.

25. Cristina Everett, "Lady Gaga Tested 'Borderline Positive' for Lupus: 'I Have to Take Good Care of Myself,'" *New York Daily News*, June 1, 2010, https://www.nydailynews.com/entertainment/gossip/lady-gaga-tested-borderline-positive-lupus-good-care-article-1.182280.

26. Christopher P. Wild and Yun Yun Gong, "Mycotoxins and Human Disease: A Largely Ignored Global Health Issue," *Carcinogenesis* 31, no. 1 (January 2010): 71–82, https://doi.org/10.1093/carcin/bgp264.

27. Lena Herden and Robert Weissert, "The Impact of Coffee and Caffeine on Multiple Scle-

rosis Compared to Other Neurodegenerative Diseases," *Frontiers in Nutrition* 5 (December 21, 2018): 133, https://doi.org/10.3389/fnut.2018.00133.

28. Kim Tingley, "The Strange Connection Between Mono and M.S.," *The New York Times Magazine*, February 23, 2022, https://www.nytimes.com/2022/02/23/magazine/epstein-barr-virus-multiple-sclerosis.html.

29. Ian C. Scott, Racheal Tan, Daniel Stahl, et al, "The Protective Effect of Alcohol on Developing Rheumatoid Arthritis: A Systematic Review and Meta-Analysis," *Rheumatology* 52, no. 5 (May 1, 2013): 856–67, https://doi.org/10.1093/rheumatology/kes376.

30. Jennifer Mannheim, "Global Increase in Rheumatoid Arthritis Prevalence Rates and Disease Burden," *Rheumatology Advisor*, October 17, 2019, https://www.rheumatology advisor.com/home/topics/rheumatoid-arthritis/global-increase-in-rheumatoid-arthritis-prevalence-rates-and-disease-burden/.

31. Adham Mottalib, Megan Kasetty, Jessica Y. Mar, et al, "Weight Management in Patients with Type 1 Diabetes and Obesity," *Current Diabetes Reports* 17, no. 10 (October 2017): 92, https://doi.org/10.1093/carcin/bgp264.

32. Marton Olbei, Isabelle Hautefort, Dezso Modos, et al, "SARS-CoV-2 Causes a Different Cytokine Response Compared to Other Cytokine Storm-Causing Respiratory Viruses in Severely Ill Patients," *Frontiers in Immunology* 12 (March 2021), https://www.frontiersin.org/articles/10.3389/fimmu.2021.629193.

33. "Long COVID (Post-Acute Sequelae of SARS CoV-2 Infection, PASC)," Yale Medicine Fact Sheet, https://www.yalemedicine.org/conditions/long-covid-post-acute-sequelae-of-sars-cov-2-infection-pasc.

34. Derek M. Griffith, Garima Sharma, Christopher S. Holliday, et al, "Men and COVID-19: A Biopsychosocial Approach to Understanding Sex Differences in Mortality and Recommendations for Practice and Policy Interventions," *Preventing Chronic Disease* 17 (July 16, 2020): 200247, https://doi.org/10.5888/pcd17.200247.

35. Katherine Mackey, Chelsea K. Ayers, Karli K. Kondo, et al, "Racial and Ethnic Disparities in COVID-19-Related Infections, Hospitalizations, and Deaths: A Systematic Review," *Annals of Internal Medicine* 174, no. 3 (March 2021): 362–73, https://doi.org/10.7326/M20-6306.

36. "COVID-19 Cardiovascular Registry Details Disparities among Patients Hospitalized with COVID," American Heart Association Scientific Sessions 2020—Late-Breaking Science, November 17, 2020, https://newsroom.heart.org/news/covid-19-cardiovascular-registry-details-disparities-among-patients-hospitalized-with-covid.

37. "People with Certain Medical Conditions," Centers for Disease Control and Prevention, May 2, 2022, https://www.cdc.gov/coronavirus/2019-ncov/need-extra-precautions/people-with-medical-conditions.html.

38. Sara Berg, "What Doctors Wish Patients New About Long Covid," American Medical Association, March 2, 2022, https://www.ama-assn.org/delivering-care/public-health/what-doctors-wish-patients-knew-about-long-covid.

39. Joseph E. Ebinger, Justyna Fert-Bober, Ignat Printsev, et al, "Antibody Responses to the BNT162b2 MRNA Vaccine in Individuals Previously Infected with SARS-CoV-2," *Nature Medicine* 27, no. 6 (June 2021): 981–84, https://doi.org/10.1038/s41591-021-01325-6.

40. Amiel A. Dror, Nicole Morozov, Amani Daoud, et al, "Pre-Infection 25-Hydroxyvitamin D3 Levels and Association with Severity of COVID-19 Illness," *PLOS ONE* 17, no. 2 (February 3, 2022): e0263069, https://doi.org/10.1371/journal.pone.0263069.

41. Christine Blume, Corrado Garbazza, and Manuel Spitschan, "Effects of Light on Human Circadian Rhythms, Sleep and Mood," *Somnologie* 23, no. 3 (2019): 147–56, https://doi.org/10.1007/s11818-019-00215-x.

42. Andrew Bartlett and Nial Wheate, "What Time of Day Should I Take My Medicine?" *The Conversation*, October 31, 2019, http://theconversation.com/what-time-of-day-should-i-take-my-medicine-125809.

43. Blume, "Effects of Light," 147–56.

44. Gregory D. Roach and Charli Sargent, "Interventions to Minimize Jet Lag After Westward and Eastward Flight," *Frontiers in Physiology* 10 (July 31, 2019), https://doi.org/10.3389/fphys.2019.00927.

45. "Data and Statistics—Sleep and Sleep Disorders," Centers for Disease Control and Prevention, September 13, 2021, https://www.cdc.gov/sleep/data_statistics.html.

46. Matt Lait, "Cave-Dwelling Volunteer Emerges 'I Love The Sun,'" *Washington Post*, May 24, 1989, https://www.washingtonpost.com/archive/politics/1989/05/24/cave-dwelling-volunteer-emerges-i-love-the-sun/af4e611f-b8af-490d-bec0-d00e638ef370/.

47. Charlotte Helfrich-Förster, Stefanie Monecke, Ignacio Spiousas, et al, "Women Temporarily Synchronize Their Menstrual Cycles with the Luminance and Gravimetric Cycles of the Moon," *Science Advances* 7, no. 5 (January 29, 2021): eabe1358, https://doi.org/10.1126/sciadv.abe1358.

48. Leandro Casiraghi, Ignacio Spiousas, Gideon P. Dunster, et al, "Moonstruck Sleep: Synchronization of Human Sleep with the Moon Cycle under Field Conditions," *Science Advances* 7, no. 5 (January 29, 2021): eabe0465, https://doi.org/10.1126/sciadv.abe0465.

49. Winnifred B. Cutler, Wolfgang M. Schleidt, Erika Friedmann, et al, "Lunar Influences on the Reproductive Cycle in Women," *Human Biology* 59, no. 6 (December 1987), 959–72, https://www.jstor.org/stable/41463960?seq=1.

50. Katherine Sievert, Sultana Monira Hussain, Matthew J. Page, et al, "Effect of Breakfast on Weight and Energy Intake: Systematic Review and Meta-Analysis of Randomised Controlled Trials," *BMJ* 364 (January 30, 2019): l42, https://doi.org/10.1136/bmj.l42.

51. Tiffany A. Dong, Pratik B. Sandesara, Devinder S. Dhindsa, et al, "Intermittent Fasting: A Heart Healthy Dietary Pattern?" *The American Journal of Medicine* 133, no. 8 (August 2020): 901–7, https://doi.org/10.1016/j.amjmed.2020.03.030.

52. Megan S. Motosue, M. Fernanda Bellolio, Holly K. Van Houten, et al, "National Trends in Emergency Department Visits and Hospitalizations for Food-Induced Anaphylaxis in US Children," *Pediatric Allergy and Immunology* 29, no. 5 (August 2018): 538–44, https://doi.org/10.1111/pai.12908.

53. Thozhukat Sathyapalan, Alireza M. Manuchehri, Natalie J. Thatcher, et al, "The Effect of Soy Phytoestrogen Supplementation on Thyroid Status and Cardiovascular Risk Markers in Patients with Subclinical Hypothyroidism: A Randomized, Double-Blind, Crossover Study," *The Journal of Clinical Endocrinology & Metabolism* 96, no. 5 (May 2011): 1442–49, https://doi.org/10.1210/jc.2010-2255.

54. Shudong He, Benjamin K. Simpson, Hanju Sun, et al, "Phaseolus Vulgaris Lectins: A Systematic Review of Characteristics and Health Implications," *Critical Reviews in Food Science and Nutrition* 58, no. 1 (January 2, 2018): 70–83, https://doi.org/10.1080/10408398.2015.1096234.

55. Stacie M. Jones, Edwin H. Kim, Kari C. Nadeau, et al, "Efficacy and Safety of Oral Immunotherapy in Children Aged 1–3 Years with Peanut Allergy (the Immune Tolerance Network IMPACT Trial): A Randomised Placebo-Controlled Study." *The Lancet* 399, no. 10322 (January 22, 2022): 359–71, https://doi.org/10.1016/S0140-6736(21)02390-4.

56. "The Current State of Oral Immunotherapy," American Academy of Allergy, Asthma & Immunology, February 4, 2020, https://www.aaaai.org/tools-for-the-public/conditions-library/allergies/the-current-state-of-oral-immunotherapy.

57. US Food & Drug Administration Office of the Commissioner, "FDA Approves First Drug for Treatment of Peanut Allergy for Children," FDA News Release, January 21, 2020, https://www.fda.gov/news-events/press-announcements/fda-approves-first-drug-treatment-peanut-allergy-children.

58. Tony Guida, "Study Finds Unsafe Mercury Levels in 84 Percent of All Fish," *CBS Evening News*, January 13, 2013, https://www.cbsnews.com/news/study-finds-unsafe-mercury-levels-in-84-percent-of-all-fish/.

59. "Arsenic," World Health Organization Fact Sheet, February 15, 2018, https://www.who.int/news-room/fact-sheets/detail/arsenic.

60. Shawn M. Burn, "What Does 'Allostatic Load' Mean for Your Health?" *Psychology Today*, October 26, 2020, https://www.psychologytoday.com/us/blog/presence-mind/202010/what-does-allostatic-load-mean-your-health.

61. Dana E. King, Jun Xiang, and Courtney S. Pilkerton, "Multimorbidity Trends in United States Adults, 1988–2014," *Journal of the American Board of Family Medicine: JABFM* 31, no. 4 (August 2018): 503–13, https://doi.org/10.3122/jabfm.2018.04.180008.

62. James Gallagher, "Child Life Expectancy Projections Cut by Years," *BBC News*, December 2, 2019, https://www.bbc.com/news/health-50631220.

63. Ibid.

64. Harvard Health Publishing, "Do You Need a Daily Supplement?" Staying Healthy, February 12, 2021, https://www.health.harvard.edu/staying-healthy/do-you-need-a-daily-supplement.

65. Claire Lampen, "Here's What's Really in the Popular Vitamins and Supplements Everyone's Taking," *MIC*, February 21, 2016, https://www.mic.com/articles/135816/here-s-what-s-really-in-the-popular-vitamins-and-supplements-everyone-s-taking.

66. Sandee LaMotte, "Just One Drink per Day Can Shrink Your Brain, Study Says." *CNN Health*, March 4, 2022, https://www.cnn.com/2022/03/04/health/alcohol-brain-shrink-age-wellness/index.html.

67. Theresa W. Gauthier, "Prenatal Alcohol Exposure and the Developing Immune System," *Alcohol Research* 37, no. 2 (2015): 279–85, https://pubmed.ncbi.nlm.nih.gov/26695750/.

68. Linda Searing, "Having a Large Waist May Mean You Are at Greater Risk of Cancer, Heart Issues, Death," *Washington Post*, March 24, 2014, https://www.washingtonpost.com/national/health-science/having-a-large-waist-may-mean-you-are-at-greater-risk-of-cancer-heart-issues-death/2014/03/24/5fde4da8-b040-11e3-9627-c65021d6d572_story.html.

69. Rebekah Honce and Stacey Schultz-Cherry, "Impact of Obesity on Influenza A Virus Pathogenesis, Immune Response, and Evolution," *Frontiers in Immunology* 10 (May 10, 2019): 1071, https://doi.org/10.3389/fimmu.2019.01071.

70. Samantha K. Brooks, Rebecca K. Webster, Louise E. Smith, et al, "The Psychological Impact of Quarantine and How to Reduce It: Rapid Review of the Evidence," *The Lancet* 395, no. 10227 (March 14, 2020): 912–20, https://doi.org/10.1016/S0140-6736(20)30460-8.

71. Amy Rushlow, "The Exact Time of Day You're Most Likely to Work Out—Successfully," *Yahoo!Life*, October 22, 2015, https://www.yahoo.com/lifestyle/the-exact-time-of-day-youre-most-likely-to-work-194319682.html.

72. "Physical Activity," World Health Organization Fact Sheet, November 26, 2020, https://www.who.int/news-room/fact-sheets/detail/physical-activity.

73. Marwa Khammassi, Nejmeddine Ouerghi, Mohamed Said, et al, "Continuous Moder-
     ate-Intensity but Not High-Intensity Interval Training Improves Immune Function Bio-
     markers in Healthy Young Men," *Journal of Strength and Conditioning Research* 34, no. 1
     (January 2020): 249–56, https://doi.org/10.1519/JSC.0000000000002737.

74. "Benefits of Physical Activity," Centers for Disease Control and Prevention, June 16,
     2022, https://www.cdc.gov/physicalactivity/basics/pa-health/index.htm.

75. José L. Areta, Louise M. Burke, Megan L. Ross, et al, "Timing and Distribution of Pro-
     tein Ingestion during Prolonged Recovery from Resistance Exercise Alters Myofibrillar
     Protein Synthesis," *The Journal of Physiology* 591, pt. 9 (May 1, 2013): 2319–31, https://
     doi.org/10.1113/jphysiol.2012.244897.

76. Goran Medic, Micheline Wille, and Michiel E. H. Hemels, "Short- and Long-Term
     Health Consequences of Sleep Disruption," *Nature and Science of Sleep* 9 (May 19, 2017):
     151–61, https://doi.org/10.2147/NSS.S134864.

77. Rebeca Gonzalez-Pastor, Peter S. Goedegebuure, and David T. Curiel, "Understand-
     ing and Addressing Barriers to Successful Adenovirus-Based Virotherapy for Ovarian
     Cancer," *Cancer Gene Therapy* 28, no. 5 (May 2021): 375–89, https://doi.org/10.1038/
     s41417-020-00227-y.

78. Judith R. Baker, Sally O. Crudder, Brenda Riske, et al, "A Model for a Regional System
     of Care to Promote the Health and Well-Being of People with Rare Chronic Genetic
     Disorders," *American Journal of Public Health* 95, no. 11 (November 2005): 1910–16,
     https://doi.org/10.2105/AJPH.2004.051318; Amy D. Shapiro, "Hemophilia B,"*NORD
     (National Organization for Rare Disorders)* (blog), https://rarediseases.org/rare-diseases/
     hemophilia-b/; J. M. Soucie, J. Symons, B. Evatt, et al, "Home-Based Factor Infusion
     Therapy and Hospitalization for Bleeding Complications among Males with Haemo-
     philia," *Haemophilia* 7, no. 2 (March 14, 2001): 198–206, https://doi.org/10.1046/j.1365-
     2516.2001.00484.x; J. M. Soucie, R. Nuss, B. Evatt, et al, "Mortality among Males with
     Hemophilia: Relations with Source of Medical Care. The Hemophilia Surveillance
     System Project Investigators," *Blood* 96, no. 2 (July 15, 2000): 437–42, https://pubmed
     .ncbi.nlm.nih.gov/10887103/.

79. Shumei Kato, Aaron Goodman, Vighnesh Walavalkar, et al, "Hyperprogressors after
     Immunotherapy: Analysis of Genomic Alterations Associated with Accelerated Growth
     Rate," *Clinical Cancer Research* 23, no. 15 (August 1, 2017): 4242–50, https://doi
     .org/10.1158/1078-0432.CCR-16-3133.

80. Cliodhna Russell, "How Often Do You Smile? Adults Only Manage 20 a Day . . .
     380 Times Less than Children," *The Journal*, July 2, 2014, https://www.thejournal.ie/
     mental-health-smile-1550017-Jul2014/.

81. Donald Lloyd-Jones, Robert J. Adams, Todd M. Brown, et al, "Heart Disease and Stroke
     Statistics—2010 Update," *Circulation* 121, no. 7 (February 23, 2010): e46–215, https://
     doi.org/10.1161/CIRCULATIONAHA.109.192667.

82. Tamar Haspel, "Perspective | The Truth about Organic Produce and Pesticides,"
     Washington Post, May 21, 2018, https://www.washingtonpost.com/lifestyle/food/the
     -truth-about-organic-produce-and-pesticides/2018/05/18/8294296e-5940-11e8-858f
     -12becb4d6067_story.html.

83. "Dietary Guidelines for Americans, 2020–2025 and Online Materials," Dietary
     Guidelines for Americans, December 2020, https://www.dietaryguidelines.gov/
     resources/2020-2025-dietary-guidelines-online-materials.

INDEX